Ketogenic

50 Delicious, Ketogenic Recipes: The Complete Guide To Going Ketogenic

By Martin Rowland

Disclaimer – Please read!

The information provided in this book is designed to provide helpful information on the subjects discussed. This book is not meant to be used, nor should it be used, to diagnose or treat any medical condition. For diagnosis or treatment of any medical problem, consult your own physician. The publisher and author are not responsible for any specific health or allergy needs that may require medical supervision and are not liable for any damages or negative consequences from any treatment, action, application or preparation, to any person reading or following the information in this book. References are provided for informational purposes only and do not constitute endorsement of any websites or other sources. Readers should be aware that the websites listed in this book may change.

Table of Contents

Introduction

Low-carbohydrate diets have been around for such a long time, yet, disputed most of the time. Primarily, fat-conscious medical practitioners have condemned the diets' principles and methodologies. Eventually, the media even joined the disapprobation bandwagon by sensationalizing to suppress completely the controversy to the public. Both sectors professed that such certain diets increase the body's cholesterol levels and result to heart ailments, obviously due to the high fat content these diets entail.

Nevertheless, this book goes along with the changing times, and enlightens you about the real essence of the ketogenic diet. There have been so many studies conducted about low-carbohydrate diets. More often than not, conclusions turned out that low-carbohydrate diets were the most favorable, compared against particular and popular diets.

Not only do they manifest increased body weight loss, but they also indicate principal improvements in most health risk factors, which include cholesterol levels. Inasmuch as they continuously provide several proven health benefits, there have been countless modified creations of the low-carbohydrate diet— and among the most accepted adaptations is the ketogenic diet.

The ketogenic diet is an exclusively low-carbohydrate, high-fat eating (LCHF) regimen, popularly practiced for the more complicated treatments of seizures. Butter, heavy cream, and vegetable oils usually provide the required fats, which fully eliminate sweets at the same time.

While other carbohydrate-rich foods have no room in the diet's strictest essence, the regimen accepts tolerances on an even more generous level. However, meals must be meticulously prepared, and accordingly measured on a weighing gram scale.

Yet, nobody really knows about the working mechanisms of the ketogenic diet, especially, on controlling seizures. Although there have been so many theories and hypotheses about how it works, the only certainty upon practicing it is the occurrence of metabolic changes that influences the chemistry of the brain. Current research, however, continues trying to unveil its mysteries thru experiments on laboratory specimens.

As such, this book will not dwell upon the diet's mechanisms of controlling seizures or epilepsy. Rather, it will be presenting you a comprehensive basic understanding about the ketogenic diet, how it efficiently works to provide a mélange of health benefits, learning about its essential food groups, and more other significant details; including, its implementation, how to start the diet, and other important tips and techniques for successfully engaging and practicing the ketogenic diet.

Furthermore, the book provides you with 50 delicious and keto-fied recipes, grouped into easy to prepare breakfast, lunch, main entrées, and side dishes. Also included are several commonly popular dishes, as well as international cuisines that presented with variations and some twists and tweaks to conform to the ketogenic diet. Exciting as it could really be, you will eventually have your shining moment to formulate your own recipes and variations soon as you get the hang of practicing your personal ketogenic diet program.

Everything you need to know now is about to unfold on each folio, until reaching the book's final canto, where you will bid adieu as a tyro, and deservingly emerge as a learned ketogenic practitioner and pro. Hereupon these pages contain all the best wishes, for you to enjoy a good read, and in the process, earn to learn something priceless!

Chapter One: What is the Ketogenic Diet?

Popularly referred to with its various monikers— keto diet, low-carb diet, low-carb / high fat (LCHF) regimen— a ketogenic diet is renowned for consuming a low-carbohydrate diet, wherein the body primarily produces chemical compounds in the liver for use as energy. Such compounds, called ketones, occur upon a shortage of insulin— a pancreatic hormone that assists the body by using glucose for energy.

Thus, with a high consumption of carbohydrates, your body produces glucose and insulin. Conversely, with low carbohydrate consumption, your body creates ketones instead.

On one hand, glucose is the most susceptible molecule converted and used as energy by your body; hence, your body easily picks it up over any other sources of energy. On the other hand, insulin, created by beta cells of the pancreas, essentially processes the glucose or the metabolism of carbohydrates. In addition, insulin regulates the glucose levels in the bloodstream by circulating it all over the body. An insufficient production of insulin results to diabetes mellitus.

Since the body principally avails the glucose and uses it as a primary form of energy, especially when having a high carbohydrate intake, your fats remain unneeded; therefore, stored anywhere else in your body. By reducing your consumption of carbohydrates and increasing the intake of fats, your body undergoes into an induced state known as ketosis.

Ketosis is a natural process, wherein your body initiates helping you survive whenever you have a low carbohydrate intake.

During the state of ketosis, the body heightens the production of ketones through the breakdown of stored fats in the liver. As such, ketosis induces the body to avail ketones for energy conversion.

Therefore, lest confusing the diet with some forms of calorie starvation, maintaining a ketogenic diet actually boils down to enforcing your body into undergoing the metabolic state of ketosis via a starvation of carbohydrates.

Indeed, nature has a way to help our bodies adapt and endure with such extremities. Upon overloading ourselves with fats and avoiding carbohydrates, our bodies has no choice left but commence burning ketones as the principal source of energy.

A History of the Ketogenic Diet

For the past thousands of years, fasting and low-carbohydrate intake, and other similar regimens related to the ketogenic diet were the predominant practices to treat certain health conditions such as, epilepsy. In fact, there was already a ketogenic diet version worked upon and recorded as early as 500 BC.

Jumping on the timeline to modern times in 1921, Dr. Rawle Geyelin presented a report to the American Medical Association, where he declared the notable beneficial results of several children after undergoing fasting. All his patients have recorded lesser seizures and other epileptic attacks, and the effects had all seemed to be enduring.

Geyelin's further research and studies continued until he developed a more acceptable low-carbohydrate and high-fat diet, now officially known as the ketogenic diet. The succeeding years have found physicians applying the diet to their epileptic patients. However, the practice had seen a drastic decline with the advent and introduction of modern anti-epileptic medications, coupled by its sensationalized reputation as a starvation regimen.

Despite the fact that the ketogenic diet has been primarily developed for the treatment of epilepsy, the diet had sparked a renewed interest during the recent past, as more and more people have recognized several medical and scientific studies that have shown proofs about the diet's numerous health and therapeutic benefits aside from the treatment of epilepsy.

Health Benefits of the Ketogenic Diet

Ketogenic diets are becoming more acceptable and favored, and for a wide variety of reasons. Established as a recommended treatment for epilepsy, along with its popular effect on losing weight, ketogenic diets are continuously under the extensive studies of medical researchers worldwide for the prevention of, and possible treatment for other neurological and health issues.

The following is a compilation from a June 2013 report of the European Journal of Clinical Nutrition about the various health conditions that ketogenic diets may overcome:

Suppress the Appetite – Eating low-carbohydrate diets and more protein and fats leads to an automatic suppression of appetite, and often end up consuming much lesser calories even without trying. Obviously, a resulting reduction in weight occurs when appetite accordingly goes down.

Weight Loss – Among the most effective and simplest ways of losing weight is cutting down on carbohydrates intake. Studies even show that individuals under a low-carb regimen tend to lose more weight much rapidly than those under low-fat diets despite the fact that the latter dieters are aggressively limiting calories.

The principal reason for this effect is that, low-carb diets impel to drain excess water from the body. Since these diets decrease the insulin levels, the kidneys begin to shed excess sodium, resulting to faster weight reduction in just a couple of weeks.

Greater Percentage of Fats Lost from the Abdominal Cavity – Fats in the body differ. Their stored location in the body determines how it affects our health. To note, the stored locations of fats are situated under the skin— subcutaneous fat; and, in the abdominal cavity— visceral fat, which tends to nestle in body organs. A high accumulation of visceral fats leads to insulin resistance, inflammation, and metabolic dysfunction.

Low-carb diets, even when compared against low-fat diets, become more effective at greatly reducing destructive abdominal fats. Moreover, a bigger percentage of those fats lost come from the abdominal cavity. With the passage of time under such a diet, the body dramatically decreases its risks to Type 2 diabetes mellitus and heart disease.

Triglycerides Favorably Decrease – Triglycerides are fat molecules in the blood, and noted risk factors for heart ailments. Low-carb diets are very effective at drastically decreasing blood triglycerides as compared to low-fat diets, where blood triglycerides tend to increase in most instances.

Increased Levels of HDL Cholesterol – High Density Lipoprotein (HDL) and Low Density Lipoprotein (LDL) indicate the lipoproteins that transport cholesterol around the bloodstream.

While LDL bears cholesterol from the liver and towards the different parts of the body, HDL moves cholesterol away from the body and towards the liver, where it may excrete or reuse cholesterol.

Since low-carb diets tend to be high in fat, they cause impressive increases in blood levels of HDL, more popularly known as the good cholesterol. Another potential indicator of heart ailment risks is the triglycerides-HDL ratio, where a higher ratio connotes greater health risks. Low-carb diets result to enhanced ratios by lowering triglycerides while raising HDL levels.

Decreasing Insulin and Blood Sugar Levels / Improving Conditions of Type-2 Diabetes – The most efficient way to lower insulin and blood sugar levels is reducing the intake of carbohydrates. In addition, a low-carb intake is a very effective way of treating, and possibly, even reversing Type-2 diabetes mellitus.

Nevertheless, when you are under current medication on lowering blood sugar levels, it is highly advised to consult with your physician prior to devising changes in your carbohydrate consumption, since your dosage may require adjustments to avoid hypoglycemia.

Decreased Blood Pressure – High blood pressure, or hypertension, is a major risk factor for many ailments, including stroke, heart disease, kidney failure and more. Studies have shown that reducing carbohydrate consumptions causes significant reduction in blood pressure, and thereby, reduced risks of several common diseases.

Treatment for Metabolic Syndrome – The metabolic syndrome is a collection of the following symptoms:

- Abdominal obesity,

- High blood pressure,

- Increased blood sugar levels,

- High levels of triglycerides; and,

- Low HDL levels

With a low-carb diet, it effectively alters and reverses all the aforementioned symptoms greatly related to heart disease and diabetes risks.

Improve Size Patterns of LDL Cholesterol – People having high levels of LDL, commonly known as the bad cholesterol, are more prone to undergo heart attacks.

However, what matters most is the type of LDL, particularly the size of its particles. Individuals having mostly smaller particles incur higher risks of heart disease, while people with mostly larger particles entail lower risks.

Studies show that low-carb diets enhance the sizes of LDL particles from small to large, and at the same time, reducing the amounts of LDL particles in the bloodstream.

Therapy for Several Brain Disorders – Our brain importantly needs glucose, but only some parts of the brain burn glucose into energy. However, a greater part of the brain can also burn ketones. This is the working principle behind the ketogenic diet, applied for quite a long time now in the treatment of epilepsy, especially when patients are unresponsive to drug treatment.

Other Possible Applications – Further medical studies declare that the ketogenic diet effectively treats many rare metabolic diseases. There have been case reports indicating its possible treatment for a certain type of brain tumor—astrocytomas. In other smaller case studies, the diet has improved conditions of type 2 diabetes mellitus, autism, migraine headaches, depression, and polycystic ovary syndrome.

Furthermore, unregulated clinical tests had shown evidences that the ketogenic diet can provide modifications in the activity of disease symptoms in a wider scope of neuro-degenerative problems, such as Alzheimer's disease, amyotrophic lateral sclerosis, and Parkinson's disease.

Whereas, the brain's glucose metabolism is impaired in Alzheimer's disease, neurological studies invoke suggestions that ketone bodies may offer an alternative energy source for the brain.

Thus, the ketogenic diet may also be a protective mechanism in strokes and traumatic brain injuries. Since tumor cells are ineffective to burn ketones for energy, the ketogenic diet is also recommendable as a treatment for cancer, like glioma brain tumor.

Although a 2013 medical review stated that, ketogenic diets provided sufficient suggestions of possible benefits to cancer therapy, the only proof of benefit at present is anecdotal.

Nevertheless, devising effective tests to measure the effects of applying a ketogenic diet in cancer treatment can be challenging.

The Diet Itself

As a review, the working principle of the ketogenic diet is essentially allowing our bodies to enter a metabolic state of ketosis.

Our bodies avail and depend upon the energy obtained from glucose, produced from our normal to high-carbohydrate consumptions. However, when there are restricted supplies of glucose— limited carbohydrates— our metabolism shifts into a fat utilization process, wherein the liver begins producing ketones.

This metabolic condition— ketosis— may appear in various forms, such as starvation, alcoholism and Type-1 diabetes mellitus. It is a state when the body's fat-burning rate is extremely high. Ketones in our blood begin to rise during this state.

Ketones may increase blood acidity that leads to some critical conditions, and thus, it is obvious that starvation is ill advised. When left unchecked, ketosis may affect urine, and result to serious kidney and liver failure.

Yet, when performed properly and responsibly, the ketogenic diet is very much effective for treating several health problems. This is the ideal condition known as optimal ketosis.

Measuring Ketones

Urine samples can measure the amount of ketones through the traditional spot test of using dipsticks, purchased from pharmacies. A dipstick, chemically coated to distinguish reactions, changes its color as it reacts with the presence of ketone bodies when dipped in a urine sample.

The presence of ketone bodies in the urine signifies the body's utilization of fat for energy instead of glucose, since insulin is not sufficiently available of using glucose to convert it into energy.

However, there are now relatively priced gadgets to measure ketone levels, though they require a prick of a needle on a finger. Within seconds, blood ketone levels are already determined.

Performing measurements are ideal with an empty stomach, preferably before breakfast. The following are the guidelines in interpreting various results of measurement values:

Lesser than 0.5-mmol/L – indicates a level which is way beyond optimum fat-burning, and it is not considered as in a state of ketosis.

Within 0.5 to 1.5-mmol/L – considered under light nutritional ketosis, it signifies receiving better effects in weight, but not in optimum conditions.

Around 1.5 to 3-mmol/L – are recommendable levels for maximum weight reduction, and the ideal state of reaching optimum ketosis.

Greater than 3-mmol/L – are negligible values since they denote achieving neither better nor worse outcomes than the recommendable levels. Sometimes, greater values may also connote that the body is not consuming enough food.

Ketogenic Diet Food Groups

Fats and Oils

Fats will be the principal source of a daily calorie intake under a ketogenic diet. Hence, choices shall conform to the digestion system in mind. While fats are essential to our bodies, they may also pose as risks when we consume the wrong types of fats.

Saturated and monounsaturated fats are chemically stable like, avocado, butter, coconut oil, egg yolks, and macadamia nuts. Such fats are more preferred since they are less inflammatory to most people.

Shy away from hydrogenated lards, like margarine, in order to minimize trans-unsaturated fat consumption. Besides, studies have linked these fats to higher risks of heart disease. When using vegetable oils like, flax, olive, safflower or soybean, select the cold- pressed types whenever available.

Thus, always opt for non-hydrogenated fats like, ghee liquid butter, beef tallow, or coconut oil. These fats have higher smoke points than other oils and allow lesser oxidization, thereby, providing more essential fatty acids.

Your meals may combine oils and fats into many different ways; either in dressings or sauces, or simply topping butter on cooked meat. Just be cautious about consuming nut or seed-based oils— almond oil, flaxseed oil, sesame oil, and any nuts other than macadamia and walnuts— since they are positively high in inflammatory Omega-6.

Carbohydrates

What chiefly determines a diet as ketogenic is the value of the consumption of carbohydrates, including a person's own body metabolism and level of activity. Generally, a diet is considerably ketogenic when it has a daily composition of less than 50 or 60 grams of net or effective carbohydrates.

However, individuals with healthy metabolisms are able to consume more than 100 grams of net carbohydrates daily, yet, retain good levels of ketosis, while older people with Type-2 diabetes mellitus may have to consume less than 30 grams net to obtain similar levels.

Protein

As you primarily reduce the carbohydrates in your diet, it does not appear as if the quantity of protein you consume is as necessary to ketosis as it often becomes eventually.

For instance, individuals under the Atkins diet— another popular weight-loss system based on a high-protein, high fat, and low-carbohydrate diet— often consume large quantities of protein during the early phases and remain under the state of ketosis.

However, most people must need to be extra cautious about the quantities of protein they consume over time, since their bodies will be adaptable with protein conversion into glucose, or gluconeogenesis. During this stage, people should test to find out whether or not too much protein is moving them away from ketosis, and make the necessary adjustments.

The best selection of protein options in a ketogenic diet is opting for anything organic or grass-fed poultry, livestock, and aquamarine produce. Organic produce reduces the consumption of steroid hormone and bacteria.

Table-1 Ketogenic Diet Protein Source

Quantity	Ketogenic Diet Protein Source	Calories	Net Carbs grams	Protein grams
6 grams	Bacon, 1 medium slice, cooked	40	0.0	2
1 ounce	Beef, Sirloin Steak, broiled	77	0.0	8
1 ounce	Beef, Ground, 4% fat, broiled	34	0.0	7.5
1 ounce	Beef, Ground, 15% fat, broiled	80	0.0	6.1
1 ounce	Beef, Roast, baked	67	0.0	8
1 ounce	Chicken, white meat	33	0.0	7
1 ounce	Chicken, dark meat	40	0.0	7
1 / 50 g	Egg, large (free-ranged)	75	0.4	6.3
1 / 56 g	Egg, extra-large (free-ranged)	81	0.4	7
1 / 63 g	Egg, jumbo (free-ranged)	90	0.5	7.9
1 ounce	Fish, Cod	30	0.0	6.5
1 ounce	Fish, Flounder	27	0.0	5
1 ounce	Fish, Sole	27	0.0	5
1 ounce	Fish, Salmon	60	0.0	7

1 ounce	Ham, smoked	40	1.0	5.3
1.25 ounce	Hot dog, beef	148	1.8	5
1 ounce	Lamb, ground	80	0.0	4.7
1 ounce	Lamb chop	70	0.0	7
1 ounce	Pork chop	60	0.0	7
1 ounce	Pork, roast	60	0.0	7
1 ounce	Pork ribs, spareribs, roasted	116	0.0	8
1 ounce	Scallops	23	2.0	6
1 ounce	Shrimp	26	1.0	6
1 ounce	Tuna	32	0.0	6.5
1 ounce	Turkey Breast	30	1.0	7
1 ounce	Veal, roasted	45	0.0	8

Vegetables – Vegetables are extremely important in the composition of any healthy diet. However, some vegetables have high sugar contents and do not fit nutritionally. Organically grown above ground vegetables are the best for a ketogenic diet. They are dark and leafy greens, and particularly high in nutrients while low in carbohydrates.

While both organic and non-organic vegetables may have the same nutritional values and properties, organically- based vegetables are much preferred to avoid pesticide residues.

Table-2 Ketogenic Diet Vegetable Source

Quantity	Ketogenic Diet Vegetable Source	Calories	Net Carbs grams	Protein grams
½ cup	Asparagus, cooked	20	2.0	2.0
3.5 ounces	Avocado	167	1.8	2.0
1/2 cup	Broccoli, chopped, cooked,	27	3.0	1.9
3.5 ounces	Carrots, raw	35	5.3	0.6
1 cup	Cauliflower, cooked	34	1.9	2.9
2 ounces	Celery, raw	9	0.7	0.4
1 ounce	Cucumber, raw	4	0.9	0.2
1 clove / 3 g	Garlic	4	0.9	0.2
½ cup	Green beans, cooked,	22	2.9	1.2
1 ounce	Mushrooms, button, raw	6	0.6	0.9
½ cup	Onion, green, chopped	16	2.3	0.9
½ cup	Onion, white, chopped, raw	32	6.0	0.9
1 ounce	Pepper, sweet, green, raw	6	0.8	0.2
1 ounce	Pickles, dill	7	1.0	0.3
1 ounce	Romaine lettuce	5	0.3	0.3
1 ounce	Butterhead lettuce	4	0.4	0.4
1 ounce	Shallots, raw, chopped	20	4.0	0.7
½ cup	Snow peas, cooked	34	3.4	2.6

5 oz	Spinach, raw	33	2.0	4.0
1 cup	Squash, acorn, baked, cubes	115	21.0	2.3
1 cup	Squash, butternut, baked, cubed	82	15.0	1.8
1 cup	Squash, summer, cooked, sliced	41	4.8	1.8
1 cup	Squash, spaghetti, cooked	42	8.0	1.0
1 ounce	Tomato, raw	5	0.7	0.2

Dairy Products – As much as possible, dairy sources of a ketogenic diet are preferably raw and organic.

Table-3 Ketogenic Diet Dairy Source

Quantity	Ketogenic Diet Dairy Source	Calories	Net Carbs grams	Protein grams
8 ounces	Buttermilk, low-fat	98	12.0	8.0
1 ounce	Cheese, Blue	100	0.7	6.0
1 ounce	Cheese, Brie	95	0.1	5.9
1 ounce	Cheese, Cheddar	114	0.4	7.0
1 ounce	Cheese, Colby	112	0.7	6.7
1 ounce	Cheese, Cottage, 2%	24	1.0	3.4
1 ounce	Cheese, Cream, block	97	1.2	1.7
1 ounce	Cheese, Feta,	75	1.2	4.0
1 ounce	Cheese, Gjetost	132	12.0	2.7
1 ounce	Cheese, Monterey Jack	106	0.2	6.9

1 ounce	Cheese, Mozzarella, whole milk	85	0.6	6.3
1 ounce	Cheese, Parmesan, hard	111	0.9	10.0
1 ounce	Cheese, Swiss	108	1.5	7.6
2 Tbsp	Cream, half-n-half	39	1.2	0.9
2 Tbsp	Cream, heavy	104	0.8	0.6
2 Tbsp	Cream, Sour, full fat	46	0.7	0.5
2 Tbsp	Cream, light whipping	88	0.9	0.7
1 ounce	Crème Fraiche	103	0.9	0.7
1 ounce	String cheese snack	80	1.0	6.0
8 ounces	Milk, whole	149	11.7	7.7
8 ounces	Milk, 2%	122	11.7	8.0
8 ounces	Milk, skim	83	12.2	8.3
8 ounces	Eggnog, full fat	224	20.5	11.6

Beverages – Dehydration is a common occurrence when undergoing a ketogenic diet since the regimen produces a natural diuretic effect. So, whether or not you are prone to bladder pains or have urinary tract infections, you must be prepared to take plenty of liquids to keep hydrated. However, be careful with liquids using sweeteners as they can contain carbohydrates.

Sweeteners – It is always prudent restricting yourself from anything sweet. The restriction tends curbing your cravings. Rather opt for artificial sweeteners when you ought to have something sweet. Choose liquid sweeteners since they do not have extra binders like dextrose and maltodextrin that contain carbohydrates.

Table-4 Ketogenic Diet Recommended Sweeteners

Sweetener	Net Carbs (Per 100g)	Calories (Per 100g)
Aspartame	85	352
Erythritol	5	20
Stevia	5	20
Sucralose	0	0
Xylitol	60	240

Nuts and Seeds

Nuts and seeds are excellent in a ketogenic diet, especially when roasted to remove anti-nutrient components. They are, however, high in Omega-6 fatty acids. Thus, consumption must be regulated.

Almonds, macadamias, pecans, and walnuts are ideal in terms of carbohydrate values. Nut and seed flours like milled flax seed and almond flour, can be great alternatives for regular flour.

While the keto diet prohibits nothing about nuts, a proper intake balance and careful monitoring is necessary for the consumption of nuts with higher carbohydrate counts, such as pistachios, chestnuts, and cashews.

Table-5 Ketogenic Diet Nuts and Seeds Source

Ketogenic Diet Nuts and Seeds Source, dry-roasted (1 ounce)	Calories	Net Carb gram	Protein gram
Almonds	161	2.9	6.0
Brazil Nuts	184	1.3	4.0
Cashews	155	8.4	4.3
Chestnuts, European	60	13.6	0.9
Chia Seeds	139	1.7	4.0
Coconut, dried and unsweetened	185	2.0	2.0
Flax Seeds	150	0.5	5.0
Hazelnuts	176	2.3	4.0
Macadamia Nuts	201	1.5	2.0
Peanuts (considered, although it is a legume)	166	3.8	6.7
Pecans	193	1.1	2.7
Pine Nuts	188	2.7	3.8
Pistachios	156	5.8	6.0
Pumpkin Seeds	163	2.2	8.5
Sacha Inchi Seeds (Inca peanut)	190	2.2	9.4
Sesame Seeds	161	2.6	4.8
Sunflower Seeds	165	3.7	5.5
Walnuts	183	1.9	7.0

Spices – This food group can be critical in ketogenic diet foods. Spices contain carbohydrates, so it is wise to consider their values.

In addition, most pre-made spice mixes have sugars added in them, so it is also better to note their nutrition labels. For salts, sea salt shall be more desired than table salt, as commonly combined with powdered dextrose.

Food list to avoid

It is always inevitable to include inconspicuously or carelessly some foods into ketogenic diets, thinking that they valuably contribute towards the diet's requirements. Therefore, hereunder is a list of foods that you must be careful:

Spices - As earlier mentioned, spices contain carbohydrates. However, there are particular spices that contain more carbohydrates than others do, such as allspice, bay leaves, cardamom, cinnamon, garlic powder, ginger, and onion powder.

Peppers – Incredible as it may seem, these little pungent and hot condiments contain sugars. So, watch out for them in stir-fried and chili-based food preparations. Choose green peppers instead, since the yellow and red varieties contain higher carbohydrate values.

Fruits – Due to their high sugar contents (fructose), ketogenic diets exclude fruits. However, their consumption is still possible for as long as following regulated portioning intakes.

Tomato-based Products – Known to be healthful, tomatoes are loaded with sugar when processed to be packaged or canned, like tomato sauces and diced tomatoes. Thus, be aware on your required portion sizes on their nutritional value labels. Sometimes, food companies are crafty to mislead nutritional values of serving sizes to make their products appear healthier.

Diet Soda – The keto diet does not really prohibit drinking diet soda since liquids are required for their hydrating purposes. Just be wary with the quantities you drink and bigger intakes of artificial sweeteners from sodas.

Medicine – Certain medications, either generic or branded over the counter drugs, like cough syrups, colds and flu medicines, generally contain carbohydrates in large amounts. Beware of these medications, as there are available low-sugar and sugar-free alternative drugs.

Chapter Two: Implementing the Ketogenic Diet

The ketogenic diet may be a medical nutrition therapy, crucially involving participants from differing disciplines. The team participants may include a registered dietitian coordinating with the diet's regular program; a registered nurse familiar with the cause and effects of the diet; and, a neurologist experienced in prescribing the ketogenic diet.

Further assistance may be availing the services of a certified medical social practitioner working with the family, and a registered pharmacist advising upon the carbohydrate values and content of prescribed medicines. Finally, for its safe implementation, immediate members of the family and other caregivers must have the necessary knowledge about the several aspects of the diet.

Implementing the ketogenic diet may pose difficulties for caregivers, as well as to the patient or practitioner due largely to the time devoted and spent regarding the planning and measuring of meals. As it is always the case, any meal unplanned may possibly break the momentum of the regular requirements of nutritional balance.

However, just as achieving success in every discipline, one requires determination and discipline. Besides, just as any aspect in educating, training, and implementing, the difficulties are always only at the beginning. On hindsight, it is just simply reciting your ABC and counting 123!

Understanding the Diet

The aim of a ketogenic diet is allowing the body to accumulate ketones through undergoing a state of ketosis. Therefore, it is noteworthy not to overdo proteins, since high-protein consumptions prevent the body from going into ketosis.

In addition, as ketosis may link itself to fasting or starvation, do not confuse the ketogenic diet as a form of intermittent fasting, which is completely another different discipline of dieting.

To enhance the production of ketone bodies, there should be reduced quantities of insulin in the bloodstream. Lower insulin levels mean sufficiently large amounts of ketone production, which is relatively the maximum effect when taking a low-carbohydrate diet.

Additionally, for the diet to be most effective, it requires the consumption of every food in its entirety. Whereas, the traditional low-carbohydrate diet comprises of ratios (in grams) of protein and carbohydrates (fat to non-fat) of 3:1 and 4:1, ketogenic diets commonly have ratios of 1:1 and 2:1.

As ketogenic diets take many forms, it typically consists of daily carbohydrate restrictions not exceeding 50 grams. Foods should relatively derive from vegetables, dairy, nuts, etc. Avoid refined carbohydrates, and refined sugars.

Thus, food must contain mostly healthy fats and protein. Ideally, the rule of thumb to follow is the 60-35-5 formula, where 60% of calories come from fat, 35% from protein, and 5% from carbohydrates. Protein must be set at 1.5 to 1.75 g for every kilogram of your ideal body weight. As a comparison, a common Western regimen comprises about 65-85% of carbohydrates, 10-20 % fat, and 5-15% protein.

Achieving Optimal Ketosis

Many practitioners of a strict low-carb regimen are often surprised to find out that their blood ketone levels are way beyond the ideal numbers. Why is this so?

The formula is not only avoiding all carbohydrate-derived foods, but also being cautious with the intake of protein. Eating large amounts of protein allows the body to convert the excess proteins into glucose.

Besides, a massive protein intake may increase insulin levels that compromise the occurrence of optimal ketosis. As a resolve, it is usually recommendable to satisfy eating with more fats. Odd as it may seem, it creates wonders though.

For instance, when having a bigger serving of butter on a steak, you quash chances or even thoughts of taking another helping of steak. Instead, you will fully have your fill after having the first serving of steak.

Another popular example of a formulaic style of ingesting more fats that is worth mentioning is taking the noted Magic Bullet Coffee (MBC) or fat coffee, where the brew uses a tablespoon each of coconut oil and butter, and blended for the proper texture.

In principle, the intake of more fats enables you to be more full, and thereby, ensuring lesser protein and carbohydrate intakes. Insulin levels will surely drop, and eventually, the body achieves optimal ketosis. Moreover, it will address overweight issues.

Experiencing the optimum hormonal effects from taking a low-carb regimen is being under the state of optimal ketosis for a prolonged duration. While under the condition of ketosis and no reduction in weight happens, it is then certain that carbohydrates are not included in the weight issue, and are not the problems to weight loss. It is noteworthy that there are other causes for obesity, and of being overweight.

Starting the Diet

When planning to start a ketogenic diet, close supervision from your medical adviser is highly necessary. Heed the cautionary advices on the ketogenic diet due to the risk of complications during the initiation of a ketogenic diet.

For instance, when you have acquired Type-1 diabetes mellitus, do not heed the aforementioned advice on optimal ketosis, as it may pose further harm on your health. Nevertheless, if ketones are indeed present in your blood, ensure your blood sugar must be at normal levels.

A normal blood sugar level is under normal ketosis, just as the ketosis possessed by healthy individuals who practice a strict low-carb regimen. On the other hand, a high blood sugar level with high blood ketones demonstrates that insulin levels are pathologically low.

Although non-diabetics do not actually suffer from these risky levels, this condition may result to ketoacidosis, or diabetes acidosis, which is a possible life-threatening situation. When this occurs, the body requires more insulin injections.

However, it is always better to consult a medical expert when you are never certain at all. Coveting high blood ketones for weight control is not worth the risk for Type-1 diabetics.

15 Top Tips for Success

While it is not necessary monitoring your daily intake of carbohydrates and calories, it definitely helps knowing exactly what you are consuming in order for you to point out easily missteps along the way. It would be more beneficial to learn a few tips towards your success in engaging with the ketogenic diet:

1. Avoid processed and canned foods if you can. Obviously, you are always unsure of their origins, derivations, and compositions, not to mention their unhealthy and diminished nutritional values.

2. Always remember the recommended and appropriate items for each food group. In this way, it facilitates you knowing what foods are necessary for consumption and those to avoid.

3. Know your macros or macronutrient consumptions. These consumptions include the three major nutrients— protein, fats, and net carbohydrate intake. Net carb consumption is your total dietary carbohydrates less your total fiber intakes. Being aware of your macros allows you to gauge the quantities of calories you need to consume, together with the proteins, fats, and carbohydrates in order to meeting your goals and achieving a successful ketogenic diet.

4. Be aware of your activity levels. It provides you with a more realistic perspective at the average quantities of calories, which your body requires to burn daily.

5. Be selective with your goals and only always apply a 10 to 15% calorie surplus or a 20 to 25% calorie deficit. Based upon studies, exceeding such deficit values may incur negative impacts regarding your dieting.

6. While a keto diet is a great way to build up muscles, you must understand that protein intake is the key and responsible for growing muscles and strengthening tissues. Thus, if you are planning to gain muscular mass, you must consume about 1.0 to 1.2g of protein per lean pound of your body weight.

7. A keto diet is not associated with a high fat consumption that causes various health problems. Rather, it is a high fat and high carbohydrates intake, which is always the culprit. Nevertheless, always consult with your physician about your concerns of the ketogenic diet.

8. About sugar cravings, medical studies have evidences connecting them to artificial sweeteners. So, when using hefty amounts of artificial sweeteners or drinking diet sodas, try skipping them altogether and modify your eating habits, lifestyles and philosophies.

9. There is truly no real harm involving yourself in a ketogenic diet lest you have a history of health issues concerning your kidney or acquiring Type-1 diabetes. Only ensure knowing that the first few days along the diet usually provide you some severe headaches and lethargic moods and movements as your body begins to adapt to the discipline.

Allow a few weeks to get the hang of it, especially its initial hump, and certainly, you will curb your usual cravings for carbohydrates.

10. It has been a common misconception that a ketogenic diet seems to be expensive. Upon seeing a low-carbohydrate diet, people will be thinking and estimating the high costs of meat. Fortunately, this is an erroneous perspective since a ketogenic diet focuses moderately on protein and more on fats, which allows more savings by emphasizing primarily on the fats.

11. Once focused starting on a healthier and more realistic approach of losing body fat, indulging in a low carbohydrate diet and lifestyle is worthwhile. The key to success concerning any diet is preparing your food in advance, or, simply creating a meal plan. A definite guideline keeps you focused and not veering away from your objectives, as well as the purposes of the diet itself.

12. While wanting to keep your carbohydrates restricted, your inclination of food consumption must principally come from dairy, nuts, and vegetables. Most of your meals must comprise proteins with vegetables, including ample amounts of fats.

13. When you find yourself famished throughout your day, try curbing your appetite by snacking out on peanut butter, cheeses, seeds, and nuts. Snacks are also part of your meal plan, and ought to be under regulation.

14. Getting quickly into a ketogenic state is dependent upon your food consumption. You must be restrictive on your

carbohydrates consumption, which only allows you less than 15g daily.

15. To maximize your results under a ketogenic diet, achieve undergoing optimal ketosis. However, this is not recommendable for individuals suffering from Type-1 diabetes. The trick here is to not only restrict you from partaking carbohydrates, but also be aware of your protein intake. The secret, unbelievably, is having your fill with lots of fats!

Shopping Guide for the Ketogenic Diet

When getting started on a ketogenic diet and you are unsure of where to take off concerning about what to take, the following shopping list below comprise the most noted ketogenic foods. The low-carbohydrate list, outlined under major food groups, is by no means extensive. Yet, it directs you towards the right path and staying on course.

It is a prudent advice to better stick to consuming mostly real and fresh foods. Real foods mean unprocessed, organic, and natural foods. While canned or processed may be beneficial in a pinch, especially when you want to take anything quick with low carbohydrate contents, it is always much healthier taking foods in their most natural form.

Meats and Poultry:
- Bacon, ham and sausage
- Beef or pork loins, ribs, ground, chops, steaks, roasts and tips
- Chicken or Turkey, whole or parts or ground

This would include any cut or type of meat; but for healthier options, opt for free-ranged, organic, and grass-fed meats, avoiding those with grain, pesticide and antibiotic residues.

Deli Meats:
- Cold cuts, like pastrami and turkey breast
- Pepperoni slices or sticks
- Prosciuttos
- Bologna and Salami

Seafood:
- Crab
- Fresh or canned salmon
- Fresh or frozen fish, scallops,
- Fresh or frozen, easy-to-peel shrimp
- Tuna in oil or water

This would include any type or kind of seafood; best options are preferably wild farmed or caught since fat levels of Omega-3 are higher.

Dairy Products
- Butter
- Cheese (hard) like parmesan and cheddar
- Cheese (soft) like farmer's and Muenster
- Cream cheese
- Eggs
- Full-fat or plain Greek yogurts, with carbohydrate counts of not more than seven per serving
- Heavy cream
- Sour cream

Low-Carbohydrate Vegetables
- Bell peppers
- Broccoli

- Cabbage
- Cauliflower
- Cucumbers
- Leafy green vegetables, as kale and spinach
- Lettuce
- Onions and garlic
- Sprouts, Brussels or kale
- Summer squash, as zucchini

Pantry
- Bottled/packed low-carbohydrate vegetables: green beans, greens, okra, and sauerkraut, with no added sugars
- Broth/Stock: chicken or vegetable
- Canned anchovies, crab, salmon, sardines, shrimp, and tuna
- Canned processed meats: luncheon meat, Vienna sausage
- Canned vegetables: artichoke hearts, chipotle peppers, green chilies, hearts of palm, mushrooms, roasted red peppers, and sun-dried tomatoes in oil
- Nut butters: natural or unsweetened (keep refrigerated upon opening)
- Sauces: Alfredo, pasta, and pizza, with no added sugars or thickeners
- Tomato products: canned tomato paste and tomatoes

Nuts and Seeds
- Nuts: almonds, hazelnuts, macadamias, pecans, and walnuts
- Seeds: sunflower, pumpkin and sesame seeds

Fruits
- Avocados: great snack with lemon juice or balsamic, or make guacamole for dipping low-carb veggies

- Eat fresh fruit with a fat such as, peanut butter, whipped cream, or cheese. It slows down spikes of blood sugar.
- Fruits are optional and depend upon a stabilized health and weight. While some people cannot handle fructose, others can and remain slim and healthy. When indulging with fruits, opt for fresh local fruits in season, and prefer sticking to typically low-sugar content fruits like, berries.

Condiments
- Capers
- Cider and wine vinegars (use balsamic vinegar sparingly)
- Horseradish
- Lemon or lime juice (1 gram of carb per tablespoon)
- Mayonnaise (seek brands with the lowest carbohydrate contents)
- Most bottled hot sauces (like sriracha, sambal oelek, Tabasco)
- Most salsas
- Mustard (except sweetened mustards like, honey mustard)
- Olives
- Sugar-free dill pickles or relish: use for tuna or egg salad
- Sugar-free salad dressings
- Tamari soy sauce (when gluten sensitive, avoid soy sauce)

Cooking or Baking Ingredients
- Almond flour or other nut flours and flour substitutes; store in freezer
- Broth or bouillon
- Cocoa powder (unsweetened)
- Erythritol, Xylitol and other sugar alcohol sweeteners
- Extracts (vanilla, lemon, almond, etc.) – avoid the ones with sugar.
- Extra-virgin olive oil
- Gelatin (plain)

- Herbs and spices (ensure to be sugar-free)
- Peanut oil and coconut oil for cooking
- Sesame oil for salad dressings
- Splenda or other artificial sweeteners like Swerve®
- Whey protein powder, plain, vanilla and chocolate flavors
- Xanthan gum for thickening and binding

Miscellaneous
- Beef jerky or beef sticks
- Pork rinds (crushed, a better alternative for bread crumbs)

Eating Out On the Ketogenic Diet

It always happens to the best of us when we have to drop by a fast food outlet or a fancied restaurant! We sometimes have no time cooking our food as we get into some tight schedules like staying late for overtime work, being busy hour after hour, becoming mobile on the road; or perhaps, getting into some other circumstances like, an out of town trip or attending parties that do not allow us preparing our own food.

As such, there will be tendencies that knock you out of the ketogenic diet and possibilities of eating foods, which you deem as right within the bounds of the dietary program, but unknowing and clueless that carbohydrates are sneakily hiding in your food's composition.

Worry not, as you can still be able to stick to your low-carbohydrate meal plan and stay on course along your dietary program by following the options and handy tips below. These may somehow help you out, making the best choice for your situation.

- It is always primordial to bear in mind to cut out on your carbohydrates. So, know the contents and values of your food.

- Prefer salads and selected fruits as your alternatives for carbohydrates.

- Always ask to verify whether served food has traces of sugar; better still, ask and check its composition prior to ordering.

- Ensure that you are not reading a menu from a soy-based vegetarian restaurant.

- Opt for places that may feed you substantially with meat or seafood; yet, be aware about their derivation, whether or not meat comes from grain or corn-fed cows or seafood fed with soy.

- When at a fast food diner, take the buns off the doggie or burger. Better, request wrapping your burger in fresh lettuce leaves, and eat it using a fork.

- Beware of noodles and pastas derived from whole-wheat grains.

- Ask olive oil or melted butter to attain or retain your ketogenic diet ratios.

- Be careful with dressings and sauces. They may contain lots of sugar. Prefer fast food chains offering salads with low-carbohydrate dressings.

- Opt for roasted, grilled, or broiled chicken over breaded or battered. When you have no options, you may peel off the skin, taking off its carbohydrates.

- When hitting the road and finding yourself hungry midst a gas station, choose filling out your tummy with deli meat, string cheese, and hard-boiled eggs, in addition to other permissible snack items such as pork rinds and almonds.

- With coffee, order an Americano, which is an espresso blended in hot water; or, a Depth Charge, also known as Turbo, Sling Blade, Shot In The Dark, and Red Eye, which is a shot of espresso blended to another drip coffee brew; in short, a double espresso. Include requesting unsweetened heavy whipping cream, coconut milk, and almonds.

Chapter Three: 10 Ketogenic Breakfast Recipes

Spinach, Sausage, and Feta Frittata

Ingredients:

12-oz	sausage
10-oz	pack frozen chopped spinach, thawed and drained
½-cup	Feta cheese, crumbled
12-pcs	eggs
½-cup	heavy cream
½-cup	almond milk, unsweetened
½-tsp	salt
¼-tsp	black pepper
¼-tsp	ground nutmeg

Directions:

1. Slice raw sausages into small pieces, and place them in a medium-sized bowl.
2. Ensure that the spinach is squeezed-dry from any remaining liquid after washing. Break the spinach up into the same bowl as the sausage.
3. Sprinkle Feta cheese over the mixture. Toss lightly until fully combined. Lightly spread the mixture onto a greased 13" x 9" casserole dish, or 18- greased muffin cups.
4. In a larger bowl, combine almond milk, cream, nutmeg, salt and pepper with the beaten the eggs together, and mix until well blended.
5. Gently pour the mixture into the dish or muffin cups until for about ¾ full.
6. Bake at 375°F for 50 minutes (for the casserole), or 30 minutes (for the muffin cups), or until fully set. Serve warm or at room temperature.

Yield: 18-muffins or 12-squares
Nutritional values per serving:
Per muffin: 137 Calories | 10g Fat | 1g Net Carbohydrates | 8g Protein
Per square: 206 Calories | 16g Fat | 1.4g Net Carbohydrates | 12g Protein

Cream Cheese Pancake

Ingredients:

2-oz	cream cheese
2-pcs	eggs
1-packet	sweetener
½-tsp	cinnamon

Directions:

1. Combine all ingredients in a blender. Blend until smooth. Allow to stand for 2 minutes for the bubbles to settle.
2. Pour ¼ of the batter into a hot pan greased with butter. Cook for 2 minutes until golden. Flip and cook 1 minute on the other side.
3. Repeat the procedure with the remaining batter. Serve with sugar-free syrup and fresh berries of choice.

Yield: 4 x 6-inch diameter pancakes
Nutritional values per serving:
344 Calories | 29g Fat | 2.5g Net Carbohydrates | 17g Protein

Scrambled Eggs with Mayonnaise

Ingredients:
50g   raw egg
23g   mayonnaise (organic)
10g   butter
Pinch of salt to taste

Directions:
1. Melt butter in a non-stick pan.
2. Using a fork, mix the egg and mayonnaise together until fully combined.
3. Cook the egg and mayo mixture in butter. Using a silicone spatula, fold gently the egg mixture until it is set.
4. Scrape the eggs and all the remaining fat onto a serving plate and serve immediately.

Yield: one serving
Nutritional values per serving:
308 Calories | 31.27g Fat | 0.53g Net Carbohydrates | 6.38g Protein

Apple and Almond Butter Cereal

Ingredients:

38g	almond butter
30g	applesauce, unsweetened
9g	coconut oil, melted
0.2 to 1 g	ground cinnamon
Pinch of salt to taste	

Directions:
1. Combine all ingredients together in a small bowl.
2. Stir well until all the ingredients are evenly integrated.
3. When the mixture is too thick, thin the consistency with water.

Yield: One serving
Nutritional values per serving:
305 Calories | 5.46g Net Carbohydrates | 8.4g Protein

Malaysian Peanut Pancakes

Ingredients:

For the roasted peanut filling

1.8-oz	fresh shelled peanuts
½-tsp	stevia
Salt to taste	

For the ketogenic condensed milk

¼-cup	heavy cream
2-drops	liquid sucralose

For the Apam Balik or turnover pancake

½-cup	almond flour
½-tsp	bicarbonate soda
½-tsp	baking powder
⅛-tsp	salt
¼-cup	almond milk
1-large	egg
5-drops	liquid sucralose
½-tsp	vanilla extract
¼-tsp	coconut oil
1-tbsp	unsalted butter

Directions:

For the roasted peanut filling

1. Preparing the peanut filling, roast 1.8 oz. freshly shelled peanuts until brown.
2. Using a pestle and mortar, grind the peanuts, ½-tsp stevia, and salt to taste. Set aside.

For the ketogenic condensed milk

3. Preparing the ketogenic condensed milk, combine heavy cream and liquid sucralose in a saucepan, and bring to a boil. Simmer and stir continuously until it thickens up like condensed milk consistency. Let cool and set aside.

For the Apam Balik or turnover pancake

4. Mix almond flour, bicarbonate soda, baking powder and salt in a bowl.
5. Add almond milk, egg, liquid sucralose, and coconut oil in the bowl, and mix well.
6. Per pancake, melt and spread ⅛-tsp coconut oil in a small pan on medium heat. Once hot, pour half of the mixture and cover the pan.
7. After the pancake is half-cooked in a minute, sprinkle half of the peanut filling.
8. Spread half of the ketogenic condensed milk onto half of the pancake, and butter onto the other half. Cover the pan again for a few minutes.
9. Remove the pancake when sides appear browned, and let cool.
10. Repeat procedures 6 to 9 for the other pancakes. Once cooled, fold the pancakes and slice to bite-sized pieces.

Yield: 2-servings
Nutritional values per serving:
539 Calories | 50.7g Fats | 6.2g Net Carbohydrates |16.1g Protein

Pumpkin Spiced-Bread French Toast

Ingredients:

4-slices	pumpkin bread
1-pc	egg, large
2-tbsps	cream
½-tsp	vanilla extract
1/8-tsp	orange extract
¼-tsp	pumpkin pie spice
2-tbsps	butter

Directions:

1. Let dry 4-slices of pumpkin bread; you may leave the slices out, uncovered overnight, achieving their desired dryness.
2. Mix egg, cream, vanilla extract, orange extract, and pumpkin pie spice in a small container.
3. Dip the bread into the mixture. Let it soak for about 5 minutes. Flip the bread and allow another 5-minute soaking.
4. Place the butter in the middle of a pan set to medium-low heat. Allow butter to cook until it begins to brown.
5. Add the soaked bread, and cook for about 3-4 minutes, or until golden brown. Flip and cook on the other side until done.

Yields: 2-servings
Nutritional values per serving:
428 Calories | 37.4g Fats | 6.8g Net Carbohydrates | 12g Protein

Cinnamon and Pecan Oatmeal

Ingredients:

1-cup	pecans, crushed
⅓-cup	flaxseed meal, ground
⅓-cup	chia seeds
½-cup	cauliflower, riced (3 oz.)
3½-cups	coconut milk
¼-cup	heavy cream
3-oz	cream cheese
3-tbsps	butter
1½-tsps	cinnamon
1-tsp	maple flavor
½-tsp	vanilla
¼-tsp	nutmeg
¼-tsp	allspice
3-tbsps	Erythritol, powdered
10-15 drops	liquid stevia
⅛-tsp	Xanthan gum (optional)

Directions:

1. Toast crushed raw pecans in a pan over low heat. Set aside.
2. Heat coconut milk in a saucepan. Add the riced cauliflower, and continue cooking until it boils.
3. Turn the heat down to medium-low, and add the seasonings: cinnamon, maple flavor, vanilla, nutmeg, and allspice.
4. Add powdered Erythritol and liquid stevia to the saucepan, and stir well.
5. Add the ground flaxseed meal and chia seeds to the saucepan and mix well. This starts to thicken the mixture.
6. Add the toasted pecans, cream, butter, and cream cheese when the mixture heats up again. Mix well. You may add Xanthan gum if you prefer the mixture to be a little thicker.
7. After a uniform consistency, remove from the heat and serve in bowls.

Yields: 6-servings

Nutritional values per serving:
398 Calories | 37.7g Fats | 3.1g Net Carbohydrates | 8.8g Protein

Cinnamon Sugar-Coated Donut Muffins

Ingredients:

For the donut muffins

1½-cups	almond flour
½-cup	Erythritol, powdered
2-tbsps	Psyllium husk powder
½-cup	heavy cream
⅓-cup	salted butter
2-pcs	eggs
1½-tsps	baking powder
½-tsp	orange extract
¼-tsp	nutmeg
¼-tsp	allspice
¼-tsp (25 drops)	liquid stevia
⅛-tsp	clove, ground
⅛-tsp	ginger, ground

For the cinnamon sugar coating

¼-cup	butter, melted
¼-cup	Erythritol or Xylitol
1-tsp	cinnamon

Directions:

For the donut muffins

1. Melt and stir occasionally salted butter in a small pan over medium-low heat.
2. Add and mix all the dry ingredients in a bowl— almond flour, powdered Erythritol, Psyllium husk powder, baking powder, nutmeg, allspice, ground clove, and ground ginger— and set aside for a moment.
3. As the melted butter smells nutty and appears golden-to-golden brown in color, set it aside or place inside the refrigerator to cool completely.
4. In a bowl, combine all wet ingredients— heavy cream, the browned and refrigerated butter, large eggs, orange extract, and liquid stevia— and beat together using a hand mixer.

5. Using a colander or strainer, sift half of the dry ingredients and combine into the wet ingredients to form the dough. Mix using a hand mixer.
6. Continue mixing the dough and combine the other half of the dry ingredients. Mix to an evenly combined dough consistency.
7. Preheat oven to 350°F. Meanwhile, measure out all the dough in silicone cupcake molds.
8. Bake for about 20-25 minutes, or until the top surfaces and edges around are golden brown.
9. Remove from the oven and set aside to cool for about 5-10 minutes.

For the cinnamon sugar coating
10. Mix cinnamon and Erythritol or xylitol.
11. Melt butter in a saucepan, and then turn the heat off.
12. Dip each muffin into the butter, including its sides and bottom. Afterwards, dip it into the cinnamon-sugar mixture. You may prefer covering only the top, or covering it entirely.

Yields: 12-donut muffins
Nutritional values per serving:
210 Calories | 20.5g Fats | 2.5g Net Carbohydrates | 4g Protein

Blackberry Pudding

Ingredients:

¼-cup	coconut flour
¼-tsp	baking powder
5-pcs	egg yolks, large
2-tbsps	coconut oil
2-tbsps	butter
2-tbsps	heavy cream
2-tsps	lemon juice
¼-cup	blackberries
2-tbsps	Erythritol
10-drops	liquid stevia

Zest of 1-pc lemon

Directions:

1. Preheat oven to 350°F.
2. Beat the egg yolks in a bowl until they appear pale in color. Add Erythritol and liquid stevia. Beat again until fully combined.
3. Add coconut oil, butter, heavy cream, lemon juice, and the zest of one lemon; beat everything together into a smooth consistency sans lumps.
4. Add the dry ingredients by sifting over the batter of wet ingredients, and then, mix well under a slow-speed mode.
5. Measure out the batter into a couple of ramekins, and distribute evenly the blackberries in the batter by lightly pushing each into the top.
6. Bake for 20-25 minutes at 350 °F. Let cool for 5 minutes or more when done.
7. To serve, pour some heavy whipping cream over the top.

Yield: 2-servings
Nutritional values per serving:
477.5 Calories | 43.5g Fats | 5.5g Net Carbohydrates | 9g Protein

Grilled Ham and Cheese Sandwich

Ingredients:
For the sandwich bread

¾-cup	almond flour
2-pcs	eggs, large
2-tbsps	coconut oil
1½-tbsps	salted butter
1-tsp	baking powder
1-tsp	coconut flour
¼-tsp	salt

For the grilled ham and cheese

3-pcs	low-carbohydrate buns
4-slices	deli ham, medium cut
1-tbsp	salted butter
2-slices	cheddar cheese
2-slices	Muenster cheese

Directions:
For the sandwich bun

1. Preheat oven to 350°F.
2. Meanwhile, mix thoroughly almond flour, salt, and baking powder in a small mixing bowl.
3. Combine butter and coconut oil into a microwave-safe container, and heat for 20 seconds or until melted.
4. Add the butter and coconut oil combination to the almond flour mixture. Mix well to make the dough.
5. Whisk the eggs and add to the dough. Continue mixing the dough.
6. Add coconut flour to thicken up the mixture and mix well.
7. Measure the dough out evenly between 8-slots in a cupcake tray by filling with a headspace of ¾-inch.
8. Bake for about 18-20 minutes, or until golden brown on the edges.
9. Remove from the oven and allow cooling prior to removing the buns from the cupcake tray.

10. Using a sharp bread knife, slice the buns into halves.

For the grilled ham and cheese
11. Place slices of deli ham in a hot pan. As they get crispy, remove them and set aside.
12. Stack the cheeses up in the following order: a slice of Muenster followed by a slice of cheddar, and repeat stacking in the same manner with the rest of the slices of cheese. Slice this stack into quarters.
13. Place a slice of cooked ham and quartered slice of cheeses in between the halved buns.
14. Melt the butter in a pan set on medium-high heat. When the butter turns brown and melted, switch the heat down to medium-low, and place the ham and cheese sandwiches. Press each sandwich on the pan.
15. Flip to cook the other side of the sandwich when the bread begins to smell slightly burnt. Allow further cooking until the top surfaces get crispy.

Yield: 8-servings of miniature buns and 8-servings of mini grilled ham & cheese.
Nutritional values per serving:
Per bun: 130 Calories | 12.3g Fats | 1.6g Net Carbohydrates | 3.8g Protein
Per grilled ham & cheese: 272 Calories | 24.2g Fats | 1.8g Net Carbohydrates | 11.3g Protein

Chapter Four: 10 Ketogenic Lunch Recipes

Bok Choy and Crispy Tofu Salad

Ingredients:
For the oven-baked tofu

15-oz	tofu, extra firm
1-tbsp	soy sauce
1-tbsp	sesame oil
1-tbsp	water
2-tsps	garlic, minced
1-tbsp	rice wine vinegar

Juice of ½-pc lemon

For the bok choy salad dressing

9-oz	bok choy
1-stalk	green onion, chopped
2-tbsps	cilantro, chopped
3-tbsps	coconut oil
2-tbsps	soy sauce
1-tbsp	sambal oelek or ground red-hot Thai chilies
1-tbsp	peanut butter
7-drops	liquid stevia

Juice of ½-pc lime

Directions:
For the oven-baked tofu

1. Press the tofu by laying them on a kitchen towel and put some heavy weight over the top, such as a cast iron skillet. Drying them out would take about 4-6 hours, so you may need replacing the towel halfway through.

2. Meanwhile, create the tofu marinade by combining soy sauce, sesame oil, water, minced garlic, rice wine vinegar, and lemon juice.
3. After drying the tofu, chop them into squares, and place in a Ziploc® bag together with the marinade. Marinate for at least half an hour, but preferably, overnight.
4. Preheat oven to 350°F. Arrange the tofu squares on a baking sheet lined with parchment paper, or a Silpat® non-stick baking mat, and bake for about 30 to 35 minutes. Set aside after cooking.

For the bok choy salad dressing
5. Mix all the ingredients except bok choy in a bowl. Mix thoroughly.
6. Chop the bok choy into small slices, as if you were to chop a cabbage.
7. Arrange the tofu and bok choy in a serving bowl, and pour the salad dressing.

Yield: 3-servings
Nutritional values per serving:
442 Calories | 35g Fats | 5.7g Net Carbohydrates | 25g Protein

Nasi Lemak (National Dish of Malaysia)

Ingredients:
For the fried chicken

2-pcs	chicken thighs, boneless
½-tsp	curry powder
¼-tsp	turmeric powder
½-tsp	limejuice
⅛-tsp	salt
½-tsp	coconut oil

For the Nasi Lemak

3-tbsps	coconut milk
3-slices	ginger
½-bulb	shallot, small
¼-tsp	salt, or to taste
7-oz	cauliflower, riced
4-slices	cucumber

For the fried egg

1-pc	egg, large
½-tbsp	unsalted butter

Directions:
For the fried chicken
1. Marinate the chicken thighs with curry powder, turmeric powder, limejuice, and salt. Let it stand for half an hour.
2. Fry the marinated chicken thighs. Set aside after cooking.

For the Nasi Lemak
3. Squeeze the riced cauliflower and drain its water out.
4. Combine coconut milk, ginger, and shallot in a saucepan, and bring to a boil.
5. Upon boiling, add the riced cauliflower, and mix thoroughly. Set aside after cooking.

For the fried egg

6. Fry the egg in melted butter. Set aside after cooking.
7. Arrange the Nasi Lemak and fried chicken over two dishes and serve with slices of cucumber and the fried egg on the side. If desired, add sambal oelek or ground red-hot Thai chilies along with the dish.

Yield: 2-servings
Nutritional values per serving:
501.7 Calories | 39.9g Fats | 6.9g Net Carbohydrates | 28.1g Protein

Sausage and Pepper Soup

Ingredients:

32-oz	pork sausage
1-tbsp	olive oil
10-oz	spinach, raw
1-pc	green bell pepper, medium, sliced
1-can	tomatoes with jalapenos
4-cups	beef stock
1-tsp	onion powder
1-tbsp	chili powder
1-tbsp	cumin
1-tsp	garlic powder
1-tsp	Italian seasoning
¾-tsp	kosher salt

Directions:
1. Cook sausage with olive oil in a large pot over medium-high heat until seared. Stir, and cook further.
2. Add sliced green pepper in the pot, and stir well; season with salt and pepper to taste.
3. Add the tomatoes with jalapenos, and stir again; and then, place the spinach on top of everything and cover the pot with its lid. When the spinach begins to wilt, add the beef broth, spices, and seasonings. Mix well.
4. Cover the pot again with its lid and cook further for half an hour, while reducing the heat to medium-low.

5. Uncover the pot and allow simmering for 15 minutes. Serve hot.

Yield: 6-servings
Nutritional values per serving:
526 Calories | 43g Fats | 3.8g Net Carbohydrates | 27.8g Protein

Almond Wrapped Lit'l Smokies®

Ingredients:

37-links	Lit'l Smokies® smoked cocktail sausage
8-oz (2-cups)	cheddar cheese
¾-cup	almond flour
1-tbsp	Psyllium husk powder
1.5-oz (3-tbsps)	cream cheese
1-pc	egg, large
½-tsp	salt
½-tsp	pepper

Directions:

1. In a microwave, melt the cheddar cheese in 20-second intervals until bubbling.
2. Remove the melted cheese from the microwave and mix it with almond flour and all the other ingredients, except the smoked sausages, to make the dough.
3. On a Silpat® non-stick baking mat, and spread the dough out until it covers the entire sheet. Place the dough in the refrigerator to harden up for about 15-20 minutes.
4. Preheat the oven to 400°F.
5. After cooling the dough, transfer it on a foil for cutting. Slice the dough into 2-inch wide by 6-inch long strips to wrap around each Lit'l Smokies® smoked cocktail sausage.
6. Bake for about 15 minutes, and then broil for a couple of minutes. Serve while hot.

Yield: 37 servings
Nutritional values per serving:
72 Calories | 5.9g Fats | 0.6g Net Carbohydrates | 3.8g Protein

Spicy Chicken Meatballs

Ingredients:
For the meatballs

1-lb	chicken meat, ground
2-tbsps	flaxseed meal
2-tbsps	almond flour
2-pcs	spring onions, medium, chopped
½-pc	red bell pepper, medium, chopped
2-tbsps	cilantro, chopped
½-tsp	garlic powder
½-tsp	salt
½-tsp	red pepper flakes

Juice and zest of ½-lime, medium

2-oz	cheddar cheese

For the guacamole dressing

1-pc	avocado, medium
¼-tsp	garlic powder

Salt & pepper to taste
Juice of ½-lime, medium

Directions:
For the meatballs
1. Preheat oven to 350ºF.
2. In a microwave, melt the cheddar cheese in 20-second intervals until bubbling. Set aside in a bowl.
3. Add all the ingredients in the bowl of melted cheddar cheese. Mix well until evenly combined.
4. Roll out the chicken mixture uniformly into meatballs. Bake the chicken meatballs for about 15 to 18 minutes, or until cooked. Set aside after cooking.

For the guacamole dressing
5. Mash the avocado by using a fork and pressing it.

6. Combine the mashed avocado with limejuice, garlic powder, and salt and pepper to taste. Mix thoroughly to a smooth consistency.
7. Serve the chicken meatballs along with the simple guacamole dressing.

Yield: 3-servings
Nutritional values per serving:
428 Calories | 31.3g Fats | 4.7g Net Carbohydrates | 33.7g Protein

BBQ Chicken Soup

Ingredients:
For the soup base

3-pcs	chicken thighs, medium
2-tsps	chili seasoning
2-tbsps	chicken fat or olive oil
1½-cups	chicken broth
1½-cups	beef broth

Salt and pepper to taste

For the BBQ sauce

¼-cup	reduced sugar ketchup
¼-cup	tomato paste
2-tbsps	Dijon mustard
1-tbsp	soy sauce
1-tbsp	sambal oelek or hot sauce
2½-tsps	liquid smoke
1-tsp	Worcestershire sauce
1½-tsps	garlic powder
1-tsp	onion powder
1-tsp	chili powder
1-tsp	red chili flakes
1-tsp	cumin
¼-cup	butter

Directions:
For the soup base

1. Preheat oven to 400°F.
2. Debone chicken thighs, and set bones aside. Season the deboned chicken thighs well with chili seasoning. Place it on a baking tray lined with foil and bake for 50 minutes.
3. Meanwhile, heat chicken fat or olive oil in a pot set on medium-high heat. Once hot, add the chicken bones, and allow cooking for at least 5 minutes.
4. Add the chicken and beef broths in the pot, and season with salt and pepper to taste.

5. Take the chicken out from the oven after cooking. Remove its skins and set them aside. Pour all of the fat from the baked chicken thighs to the broth and stir to combine.

For the BBQ sauce
6. Combine all the ingredients and mix thoroughly to produce the BBQ sauce.
7. Pour the BBQ sauce to the pot and stir to combine. Simmer for about 20 to 30 minutes.
8. Emulsify all of the fats and liquids together by using an immersion blender.
9. Shred the chicken thighs and add to the soup. You may add bell pepper or spring onion, as desired.
10. Simmer for another 10 to 20 minutes. Serve with spring onion, yellow bell pepper, cheddar cheese and those crispy chicken skins.

Yield: 4-servings
Nutritional values per serving:
487 Calories | 38.3g Fats | 4.3g Net Carbohydrates | 24.5g Protein

Cabbage and Chicken Puree

Ingredients:

100g	chicken broth
30g	raw green cabbage, shredded
5g	raw onion, diced small
1g	raw garlic, finely diced
20g	cooked chicken breast, diced
15g	butter
15g	olive oil
15g	mayonnaise

Dash of salt & white pepper to taste

Directions:

1. Add olive oil, and butter to melt, in a small pot, set over medium heat.
2. Add the cabbage, onions and garlic, and sauté until vegetables soften. Add the broth and chicken.
3. Cover the pot and allow simmering over low heat until vegetables are tender.
4. Remove the pot from the heat and add the mayonnaise. Stir well before serving.

Yield: 2-servings
Nutritional values per serving:
397 Calories | 2.5g Net Carbohydrates | 7.35g Protein

Pork Stew: Southwestern Style

Ingredients:

1-lb	cooked pork shoulder, sliced
2-tsps	chili powder
2-tsps	cumin
1-tsp	garlic, minced
½-tsp	salt
½-tsp	pepper
1-tsp	paprika
1-tsp	oregano
¼-tsp	cinnamon
2-pcs	bay leafs
6-oz	button mushrooms
½-pc	jalapeno, sliced
½-bulb	onion, medium
½-pc	green bell pepper, sliced
½-pc	red bell pepper, sliced
2-cups	gelatinous bone broth
2-cups	chicken broth
½-cup	strong coffee
¼-cup	tomato paste

Juice of ½-lime (to finish)

Directions:

1. Sauté all the vegetables with olive oil in a pan, set over high heat. Remove from the heat once the vegetables exude their aroma.
2. Place the sliced pork in a slow cooker, together with the button mushrooms, gelatinous bone broth, chicken broth, and strong coffee.
3. Add the sautéed vegetables and spices in the slow cooker, and mix well. Cover the slow cooker with its lid and allow cooking under low heat for about 4 to 10 hours.

Yield: 4-servings

Nutritional values per serving:
386 Calories | 28.9g Fats | 6.4g Net Carbohydrates | 19.9g Protein

Pasta à la Carbonara

Ingredients:

⅔-cups	pasta, cooked
5-oz	bacon
2-pcs	egg yolks, large
1-pc	egg, large
1-tbsp	heavy cream
⅓-cup	fresh grated parmesan
3-tbsps	fresh basil, chopped

Freshly ground black pepper to taste

Directions:

1. Start freezing the bacon for 15 minutes. After freezing, chop it into small cubes. Cook the cubes of bacon with its own grease until crisp. Set aside after cooking and set aside a third of its grease.
2. Combine egg, egg yolks, parmesan cheese, and the bacon grease to form the sauce. Mix well to a thick consistency.
3. Place the pasta with the remaining bacon grease in a pan set over high heat. Cook until pasta is slightly crisp.
4. Combine the pasta, sauce, bacon, freshly ground black pepper and 2-tbsps of fresh basil in a bowl. Mix thoroughly.
5. Divide into three servings and garnish with the remaining tablespoon of fresh chopped basil and freshly ground black pepper.

Yield: 3-servings
Nutritional values per serving:
553 Calories | 44g Fats | 3.8g Net Carbohydrates | 21.7g Protein

Spiced Pumpkin Puree

Ingredients:

1½-cups	chicken broth
1-cup	pumpkin puree
4-tbsps	butter
¼-bulb	onion, medium, chopped
2-cloves	garlic, minced, roasted
½-tsp	salt
½-tsp	pepper
½-tsp	ginger, freshly minced
¼-tsp	cinnamon
¼-tsp	coriander
⅛-tsp	nutmeg
1-pc	bay leaf
½-cup	heavy cream
4-slices	bacon
3-tbsps	bacon grease (from the bacon)

Directions:

1. Melt the butter until browned in a saucepan over medium-low heat. Add onions, garlic, and ginger to the pan. Cook for about 2 to 3 minutes.
2. When onions are translucent, add the spices and stir well. Cook for a couple of minutes, and then add pumpkin puree and chicken broth to the pan. Stir well.
3. Bring the mixture to a boil. Switch into low heat and allow simmering for about 20 minutes. Using an immersion blender, emulsify the broth mixture to a smooth consistency. Simmer for another 20 minutes.
4. Meanwhile, cook the slices of bacon with its own grease until crisp. Set aside after cooking.
5. After cooking the broth, add the bacon grease and heavy cream. Mix to combine well.
6. As desired, you may add chopped parsley and 2-tbsps of sour cream. Serve by crumbling the bacon over the broth.

Yield: 3 x 1-cup servings
Nutritional values per serving:
486 Calories | 48.7g Fats | 7.3g Net Carbohydrates | 5.7g Protein

Chapter Five: 20 Ketogenic Dinner Recipes

Cheesy Au Gratin Cauliflower

Ingredients:

4-cups	raw cauliflower florets
4-tbsps	butter
⅓-cup	heavy whipping cream
6-pcs	Pepper jack cheese, deli slices

Dash of salt and pepper to taste

Directions:
1. Mix all ingredients except the Pepper jack cheese in a microwave dish. Combine thoroughly.
2. Heat the cauliflower mixture in the microwave for about 25 minutes, or until tender.
3. Remove from the microwave and mash with a fork. Add more salt or pepper to taste.
4. Lay slices of cheese over the cauliflower mixture. Heat again until the cheese melts. Serve hot.

Yield: 6 x ¾-cup servings
Nutritional values per serving:
215 Calories | 19g Fat | 2g Net Carbohydrates | 6g Protein

Cheesy and Spicy Spaghetti Squash Casserole

Ingredients:
For the chili

1-lb	lean ground beef (or turkey)
1-tsp	cumin, ground
1-tsp	coriander, ground
1-tbsp	chopped chipotles in adobo (optional)
½-tsp	garlic powder
1-tsp	dried oregano
½-cup	prepared salsa

Salt and pepper to taste

For the casserole

4-cups	spaghetti squash, cooked
2-tbsps	butter, melted
¾-cup	sour cream
1¾-cups	Mexican cheese, shredded

Chopped cilantro (optional)
Sour cream, salsa, avocado to serve (optional)

Directions:
For the chili:
1. Season the ground meat with salt and pepper, and cook it in a medium-sized saucepan until browned.
2. Discard any extra fat and add the remaining chili ingredients. Simmer for about 10 minutes.

For the casserole:
3. Combine the cooked spaghetti squash and melted butter in a medium-sized bowl. Toss to coat the pasta with butter, and then, season generously with salt and pepper to taste.
4. Spread out the spaghetti squash in a 14-inch casserole dish. Sprinkle with ¾-cup of shredded Mexican cheese. Spread the sour cream over the cheese layer. Spoon on the chili and spread it out, leaving a 1-inch border of spaghetti squash

around the edge. Top with the remaining 1 cup of shredded cheese.
5. Bake at 350ºF for 30 minutes.
6. Sprinkle with cilantro and serve with sour cream, salsa, and guacamole or avocado slices, as desired.

Yield: 8 x 1-½ cup servings
Nutrition values per serving:
284 Calories | 20g Fat | 6g Net Carbohydrates | 23g Protein

Sun-dried Tomatoes and Feta Meatballs

Ingredients:

1-lb	ground turkey
¼-cup	feta cheese, crumbled
2-tbsps / 5-oz	sun-dried tomatoes, chopped
1-bsp	fresh thyme leaves (or ½-tsp thyme leaves, dried)
1-pc	egg
½-tsp	garlic powder
¼-cup	almond flour
2-tbsps	water
Olive oil for frying	

Directions:

1. Combine all ingredients except olive oil in a medium bowl. Mix well.
2. Form 1-inch diameter meatballs out of the mixture.
3. Fry meatballs in olive oil in a large sauté pan until golden brown.

Yield: 4 x 4-meatballs servings
Nutritional values per meatball:
89 Calories | 8g Fat | 0.65g Net Carbohydrates | 6g Protein

Cuban Pot Roast

Ingredients:

2.5 to 3 lbs	boneless chuck roast
½-cup	salsa verde or green sauce
½-cup	green chili, canned, chopped
1-cup	tomatoes, diced
2-tbsps	dried onion flakes
1-tsp	garlic powder
½-cup	red and yellow peppers, cut into strips
1-tsp	salt
2-tbsps	ground cumin
1-tbsp	ground coriander
1-tsp	dried oregano
1-tbsp	chili powder
½-tsp	black pepper
2 Tbsp	apple cider vinegar

Directions:

1. Season the boneless chuck roast generously with salt and pepper. Sear it in a hot pan until browned on all sides.
2. Place the meat in the bottom of a 5-quart Crock-Pot® slow cooker.
3. In the pan used to sear the meat, add the salsa verde, chili, and tomatoes. Deglaze and bring to a boil.
4. Pour the mixture over the meat in the Crock-Pot®. Add all the remaining ingredients into the slow cooker and stir thoroughly.
5. Cook for 4 hours over high heat, or 6 hours over low heat, or until the meat is tender.
6. Shred the meat and serve with toppings of your choice.

Yield: 10 x 1-cup servings
Nutritional values per serving:
271 Calories | 19g Fat | 2g Net Carbohydrates | 20g Protein

Chicken Wings in Blackberry Chipotle

Ingredients:
3-lbs (20-wings)   chicken wings, butchered
½-cup   blackberry chipotle jam
½-cup   water
Salt and pepper to taste

Directions:
1. Slice the chicken wings to separate drummettes, wings, and wing tips. Set aside wing tips for future use in bone broth.
2. Combine blackberry chipotle jam and water in a bowl to create the marinade.
3. Whisk the mixture well, and then add ⅔-marinade with the chicken wings in a Ziploc® bag. Season the marinade with salt and pepper to taste. Let it sit for at least half an hour, or overnight.
4. When ready, preheat oven to 400°F.
5. Lay chicken on a cookie sheet with a wire rack on top. Bake for 15 minutes at 400°F, then flip and turn oven up to 425°F. Brush the remaining marinade over each wing, and bake for about 20 to 30 minutes.

Yield: 5 x 4-wing servings
Nutritional values per serving:
503 Calories | 39.1g Fats | 1.8g Net Carbohydrates | 34.5g Protein

Crispy Sesame Beef on Daikon Radish

Ingredients:

1-pc (about ¾-lb)	daikon radish, medium
1-lb	rib-eye steak, sliced into ¼-inch strips
1-tbsp	coconut flour
½-tsp	guar gum
1-tbsp	coconut oil
4-tbsps	soy sauce
1-tsp	sesame oil
1-tsp	oyster sauce
1-tbsp + 1 tsp	rice vinegar
1-tsp	sriracha or sambal oelek
½-tsp	red pepper flakes
1-tbsp	toasted sesame seeds
½-pc	red pepper, medium, sliced into thin strips
½-pc	jalapeño pepper, medium, sliced into thin rings
1-pc	green onion, medium, chopped
1-clove	garlic, minced
1-tsp	ginger, minced
7-drops	liquid stevia
Oil for frying	

Directions:

1. Slice the daikon radish into noodle-like strings. Soak the radish noodles in a bowl of cold water for about 20 minutes.
2. Chop the rib-eye steak into small strips, about ¼-inch thick. Coat the strips with coconut flour and guar gum, and let them sit for 10 minutes.
3. Heat oil in a wok, and add garlic, ginger, and red pepper. Fry until aromatic. Add the soy sauce, oyster sauce, sesame oil, rice vinegar, liquid stevia and sriracha. Whisk together and cook for about 2 minutes.
4. Meanwhile, heat the cooking oil in a large pot. Add beef strips, ensuring not to overcrowd the pot. Fry the meat for about 2 to 3 minutes on each side, or until browned.

5. Place the meat on paper towels to absorb some of the oil. Put it in the wok to combine with the vegetables and sauce. Cook for another couple of minutes.
6. Drain the daikon radish noodles. Divide them onto each serving plate. Top each with sesame beef.

Yield: 4-servings
Nutritional values per serving:
412 Calories | 31.3g Fats | 5g Net Carbohydrates | 24.5g Protein

Chicken Curry

Ingredients:

2-tbsps	coconut oil
1.5-inch	ginger, pounded
1-pc	green chili, pounded
2-pcs	shallots, pounded
2-cloves	garlic, pounded
2-tsps	turmeric powder
1-stalk	lemongrass, bruised
½-cup	coconut milk
½-cup	water
21-oz	chicken
½-tsp	salt
1-tbsp	cilantro, chopped

Directions:
1. Sauté the pounded ingredients in coconut oil in a pan set on medium heat for about 3 to 4 minutes.
2. Add the bruised lemongrass and turmeric powder, and sauté again.
3. Add the chicken. Mix well.
4. Pour coconut milk and water, and salt. Mix well to combine thoroughly.
5. Cover the pan and simmer for about 20 minutes, or until the sauce thickens.
6. Sprinkle with chopped cilantro and serve.

Yield: 3-servings
Nutritional values per serving:
493 Calories | 35g Fats | 4.8g Net Carbohydrates | 37.5g Protein

Skillet Chicken Pot Pie

Ingredients:
For the filling

6-pcs	chicken thighs, de-boned and de-skinned
5-slices	bacon
1-tsp	onion powder
1-tsp	garlic powder
¾-tsp	celery seed
8-oz	cream cheese
4-oz	cheddar cheese
6-cups	spinach
¼-cup	chicken broth

Salt and pepper to taste

For the crust

⅓-cup	almond flour
3-tbsps	Psyllium husk powder
3-tbsps	butter
1-large	egg
¼-cup (2 oz)	cream cheese
¼-cup	cheddar cheese
½-tsp	paprika
¼-tsp	garlic powder
¼-tsp	onion powder

Salt and pepper to taste

Directions:
For the filling

1. Slice the chicken thighs into cubes and season with salt and pepper.
2. Place the cubed chicken thighs in an oven-safe hot pan, and season with spices. Allow cooking for a few minutes until browned on the outside.
3. Cut bacon into small pieces and place in the pan. Allow cooking until browned.
4. Preheat the oven to 375°F.

5. Use the chicken broth to de-glaze the pan, and then, add cheddar cheese and cream cheese. Mix well.
6. Add the spinach to the pan and let it wilt. Upon wilting, stir thoroughly.

For the crust
7. Place all the dry ingredients in a bowl, while the cheddar and cream cheese in another. Melt the cheese for about 30 seconds in the microwave. Add the egg and melted cheese to the dry ingredients, and mix well.
8. After mixing, form into a circle on a Silpat® non-stick baking mat. Ensure a diameter to be the same as the pan's size.
9. Carefully invert the non-stick baking mat with the crust over the pan and peel the mat off.
10. Place the pan in the oven and allow cooking for about15 minutes at 375°F.

Yield: 8-servings
Nutritional values per serving:
434 Calories | 35.6g Fats | 3.4g Net Carbohydrates | 20.4g Protein

Salmon Filet with Dill and Tarragon Cream Sauce

Ingredients:
For the salmon filets

1½-lb	salmon, sliced in half to produce 2-filets
¾ to 1-tsp	dried tarragon
¾ to 1-tsp	dried dill weed
1-tbsp	duck fat

Salt and pepper to taste

For the cream sauce

2-tbsps	butter
¼-cup	heavy cream
½-tsp	dried tarragon
½-tsp	dried dill weed

Salt and pepper to taste

Directions:
For the salmon filets
1. Season meat the salmon filets with spices, while the skin side with salt and pepper.
2. Heat the duck fat in a ceramic cast iron skillet, set over medium heat. Place the salmon filets in the skillet, with the skin side down.
3. Allow cooking for about 4 to 6 minutes until the skin is crisp. Turn to low heat, and flip the salmon to cook for about 15 minutes.
4. Remove the salmon from the pan and set aside. Add butter and spices to the pan.

For the cream sauce
5. Mix all the cream sauce ingredients well, and pour the sauce all over the salmon to serve.

Yield: 2-servings
Nutritional values per serving:
469 Calories | 40g Fats | 1.5g Net Carbohydrates | 22.5g Protein

Duck Breast Glazed in Sage and Orange

Ingredients:

1-pc (6 oz)	duck breast
2-tbsps	butter
1-tbsp	heavy cream
1-tbsp	Swerve® sweetener
½-tsp	orange extract
¼-tsp	sage
1-cup	spinach

Directions:

1. Season the duck breast with salt and pepper.
2. Add butter and Swerve® sweetener in a pan, set over medium-low heat. Cook until browned.
3. Add orange extract and sage. Cook until butter is in a deep amber color. Add heavy cream, and mix well. Set aside after cooking.
4. Meanwhile, place the duck breast in another pan, set over medium-high heat.
5. Cook and flip the duck breast until its skin is crisp.
6. Pour the orange extract and sage mixture over the duck breast in the pan, to allow blending with the duck's fat. Cook for a few minutes longer.
7. In the pan, you used to make the sauce, wilt the spinach; and then, add to combine with the duck's breast in the pan.

Yield: One serving
Nutritional values per serving:
798 Calories | 71g Fats | 0g Net Carbohydrates | 36g Protein

Rib-eye Steak

Ingredients:

1-16oz	rib-eye steak (1 to 1¼-inch thick)
1-tbsp	duck fat (or peanut oil)
1-tbsp	butter
½-tsp	thyme, chopped

Salt and pepper to taste

Directions:

1. Preheat oven to 400ºF with a cast iron skillet inside.
2. Prepare the rib-eye steak by seasoning with oil, salt and pepper.
3. After preheating the skillet, remove from oven and set over medium heat. Add oil, and then the steak in the skillet. Allow searing for a couple of minutes.
4. Flip the steak and place in the oven to roast for about 4 to 6 minutes.
5. Remove steak and place over the stove, set in low heat.
6. Add butter and thyme in the skillet, and baste steak for about 2 to 4 minutes.
7. Let it sit for about 5 minutes, and serve.

Yield: 2-servings
Nutritional values per serving:
750 Calories | 66g Fats | 0g Net Carbohydrates | 38g Protein

Roasted Turkey Legs

Ingredients:

2-pcs	turkey legs
2-tbsps	duck fat (or peanut oil)
2-tsps	salt
½-tsp	pepper
¼-tsp	cayenne pepper
½-tsp	onion powder
½-tsp	garlic powder
½-tsp	dried thyme
½-tsp	ancho chili powder
1-tsp	liquid smoke
1-tsp	Worcestershire sauce

Directions:
1. Combine all dry spices in a small bowl. Add all the wet ingredients in another bowl, and mix well.
2. Pat the turkey legs completely dry, and rub thoroughly with seasoning.
3. Preheat the oven to 350ºF.
4. Place the duck fat in a cast iron skillet, set over medium-high heat. Upon the oil starts smoking, add the turkey legs in the skillet, and sear on each side for about a couple of minutes.
5. Transfer the skillet in the oven, and roast at 350 ºF for an hour, or until cooked.

Yield: 4-servings
Nutritional values per serving:
382 Calories | 22.5g Fats | 0.8g Net Carbohydrates | 44g Protein

Chicken Parmesan

Ingredients:
For the coating

2.5-oz	pork rinds
¼-cup	flaxseed meal
½-cup	parmesan cheese
1-tsp	oregano
½-tsp	salt
½-tsp	pepper
¼-tsp	red pepper flakes
½-tsp	garlic
2-tsps	paprika
1-pc	egg, large
1½-tsp	chicken broth

For the chicken

3-pcs	chicken Breasts
1-cup	mozzarella cheese, grated

Salt and pepper to taste

For the sauce

¼-cup	olive oil
1-cup	Rao's tomato sauce
¼-cup	oil
½-tsp	garlic
½-tsp	oregano

Salt and pepper to taste

Directions:
For the coating
1. In a food processor, grind the pork rinds, flax, parmesan cheese, and spices up.
2. Whisk the egg with the chicken broth in a separate container.

For the chicken

3. Cut the chicken breasts in half or in thirds and pound them out into cutlets.
4. Bread all chicken cutlets by dipping into egg mixture, then dipping into the coating mixture. Set aside on a piece of foil.
5. Heat 2 tbsp. olive oil in a pan and fry up each piece of chicken, two at a time. Add more oil, as necessary.

For the sauce
6. Combine all ingredients for the sauce in a saucepan, and whisk well. Allow cooking for at least 20 minutes, and set aside after cooking.
7. Arrange the pieces of cooked chicken into a casserole dish, add sauce as toppings, and then sprinkle with grated mozzarella cheese.
8. Bake at 400ºF for about 10 minutes, or until cheese melts.

Yield: 4-servings
Nutritional values per serving:
646 Calories | 46.8g Fats | 4g Net Carbohydrates | 49.3g Protein

Bacon and Cheeseburger Soup

Ingredients:

5-slices	bacon
12-oz	ground beef
2-tbsps	butter
3-cups	beef broth
½-tsp	garlic powder
½-tsp	onion powder
2-tsps	brown mustard
1½-tsp	kosher salt
½-tsp	black pepper
½-tsp	red pepper flakes
1-tsp	cumin
1-tsp	chili powder
2½-tbsps	tomato paste
1-pc	dill pickle, medium, diced
1-cup	cheddar cheese, shredded
3-oz	cream cheese
½-cup	heavy cream

Directions:

1. Cook the slices of bacon in a pan until crispy. Set aside after cooking.
2. Cook the ground beef with the bacon fat until browned on one side; flip and brown the other side.
3. Transfer the beef to a pot, and arrange moving it to the sides. Add butter and spices in the pot, and allow sweating them for about a minute.
4. Add the beef broth, tomato paste, cheese, and pickles in the pot, and allow cooking for a few minutes until melted.
5. Cover the pot and switch into low heat. Cook for about 20 to 30 minutes.
6. Finish it off by adding heavy cream and crumbled bacon. Stir well and serve.

Yield: 5-servings

Nutritional values per serving:
572 Calories | 48.6g Fats | 3.4g Net Carbohydrates | 23.4g Protein

Stuffed Meatballs à la Italiana

Ingredients:

1½-lbs	ground beef
1-tsp	oregano
½-tsp	Italian seasoning
2-tsps	garlic, minced
½-tsp	onion powder
3-tbsps	tomato paste
3-tbsps	flaxseed meal
2-pcs	eggs, large
½-cup	olives, sliced
½-cup	mozzarella cheese
1-tsp	Worcestershire sauce

Salt and pepper to taste

Directions:
1. Preheat the oven to 400ºF.
2. Combine the ground beef with all of the ingredients and form into meatballs. Lay the meatballs on a foil-covered cookie sheet.
3. Place the sheet in the oven, and bake for about 20 minutes.
4. Drizzle all over with fat from the sheet.

Yield: 4-servings
Nutritional values per serving:
594 Calories | 44.8g Fats | 3.8g Net Carbohydrates | 36.8g Protein

Spicy Chicken Nuggets

Ingredients:
For the crust

1.5-oz	pork rinds
¼-cup	almond meal
¼-cup	flax meal
¼-tsp	salt
¼-tsp	pepper
¼-tsp	chili powder
¼-tsp	paprika
⅛-tsp	onion powder
⅛-tsp	garlic powder
⅛-tsp	cayenne pepper

Zest of 1-pc lime

For the chicken nuggets

24-oz	chicken thighs, sliced into bite-size pieces
1-pc	egg, large

For the sauce

½-cup	mayonnaise
½-pc	Hass avocado, medium
½-tsp	red chili flakes
1-tbsp	limejuice
¼-tsp	garlic powder
⅛-tsp	cumin

Directions:
For the crust
1. Pulse all of the ingredients for the crust in a food processor.
2. Put the crumbs in a bowl and a whisked egg in another.

For the chicken nuggets
3. Dip the chicken in the whisked egg, then in the crust. Lay the coated chicken on a greased baking sheet.

4. Place the sheet in the oven, and bake at 400°F for about 18 minutes.

For the sauce
5. Combine all the sauce ingredients, and mix well.

Yield: 4-servings
Nutritional values per serving:
613 Calories | 50g Fats | 1.8g Net Carbohydrates | 38.8g Protein

Slow-Roasted Crispy Pork Shoulder

Ingredients:

8-lbs	pork shoulder
3½-tbsps	salt
2-tsp	oregano
1-tsp	black pepper
1-tsp	garlic powder
1-tsp	onion powder

Directions:

1. Preheat the oven to 250ºF.
2. Rinse and dry up the pork. Rub salt and spices over the entire pork shoulder. Set it aside in room temperature for a few hours.
3. Place onto a wire rack sitting over a baking sheet covered in foil.
4. Bake the pork for about 8 to 10 hours, or until internal temperature is about 190ºF.
5. Cover the pork with foil, and let it sit for about 15 minutes. Meanwhile, heat the oven to 500ºF.
6. Remove the foil and roast the pork again for about 20 minutes at 500ºF, while rotating it for every 5 minutes.
7. Let it sit for about 15 to 20 minutes prior to cutting and serving.

Yield: 20 x 6-oz servings
Nutritional values per serving:
461 Calories | 36.7g Fats | 0.2g Net Carbohydrates | 30.3g Protein

Baked Chicken Thighs

Ingredients:
6-pcs	chicken thighs, bone-in, skin-on
1-tbsp	olive oil
1-tbsp	ketchup, reduced sugar
1-tbsp	rice wine vinegar
2-tsps	sriracha
1-tsp	garlic, minced
1-tsp	ginger, minced
¼-tsp	Xanthan gum

Salt and pepper to taste

Directions:
1. Preheat the oven to 425ºF.
2. Pat chicken dry, and season skin-side with salt and pepper.
3. Mix all the sauce ingredients in a small container until forming a thick paste.
4. Rub the sauce entirely over the chicken thighs.
5. Lay the chicken thighs on a wire rack over a baking sheet covered in foil.
6. Bake for about 40 to 50 minutes until skin is crisp and charring appears.

Yield: 4-servings
Nutritional values per serving:
606 Calories | 53.5g Fats | 1.5g Net Carbohydrates | 28.8g Protein

Chicken in Creamy Tarragon

Ingredients:

5-oz	chicken breast cut in cubes
1-tbsp	olive oil
¼-pc	small onion, sliced thin
3-oz	mushrooms
½-cup	chicken broth
¼-cup	heavy cream
1-tsp	grain mustard
½-tsp	dried tarragon

Salt and pepper to taste

Directions:

1. Season the chicken breast cubes with salt and pepper to taste.
2. Heat olive oil in a pan, set over medium-high heat. Add the seasoned chicken cubes to the pan and brown on each side. Set aside after cooking.
3. In the same pan, add the mushrooms, and cook until browned. Add the sliced onion and cook further until the onion becomes translucent.
4. Add the chicken broth to the pan, and switch into low heat while cooking for about 3 to 4 minutes.
5. Add the rest of the ingredients and season to taste. Mix well, and then add the cooked chicken cubes in the pan. Allow this to reduce slightly while cooking for an additional five minutes.

Yield: One serving
Nutritional values per serving:
490 Calories | 40g Fats | 5g Net Carbohydrates | 32g Protein

Bell Peppers Stuffed with Korean Beef BBQ

Ingredients:
For the meat & peppers

1-lb	ground beef
2-pcs	bell peppers, sliced in half
2-stalks	spring onions, sliced thin
2-tsps	garlic, minced
2-tsps	ginger, minced

8-pcs eggs, large
Salt and pepper to taste

For the Korean BBQ sauce

1/3-cup	apricot preserves, sugar-free
1½-tbsps	rice wine vinegar
1-tbsp	ketchup, reduced sugar
1-tbsp	chili paste
1-tbsp	soy sauce

Directions:
For the meat & peppers
1. Cook the ground beef until browned in a pan, set over medium-high heat. Season it with salt and pepper.
2. Add garlic and ginger when the beef turns brown, and mix.
3. Move the beef to one side of the pan and add sliced spring onions to fry. Allow cooking for a couple of minutes. Set aside after cooking.
4. Fry the eggs, and set them aside.

For the Korean BBQ sauce
5. Combine all the sauce ingredients in a small saucepan, set over medium heat. Cook until the mixture slightly thickens.
6. Add half of the sauce to the cooked beef.
7. Stuff each halved bell pepper with beef.
8. Bake the bell peppers for about 12 to 15 minutes at 350ºF.
9. Glaze the top surfaces of the bell peppers with the remaining sauce.

10. Serve with two fried eggs per halved bell pepper.

Yield: 4-half stuffed bell pepper servings
Nutritional values per serving:
470 Calories | 35g Fats | 6.3g Net Carbohydrates | 32.3g Protein

Chapter Six: 10 Ketogenic Side Dishes Recipes

Tater Tots

Ingredients:

1-head	cauliflower, medium, cut into florets
¼-cup	parmesan cheese, grated
2-oz	mozzarella cheese, shredded
1-pc	large egg
½-tsp	onion powder
½-tsp	garlic powder
2-tsps	Psyllium husk powder
1-cup	oil for deep-frying

Salt and pepper to taste

Directions:
1. Steam the cauliflower until tender.
2. Put the steamed cauliflower in a food processor, and pulse until it appears like mashed potatoes.
3. Place the pulsed cauliflower on a dishcloth to cool and wring out any excess water.
4. In a bowl, combine the drained out cauliflower with cheese, egg, and spices. Mix until thickened.
5. Add a teaspoon of Psyllium husk powder at a time to the mixture.
6. Create tater tots by rolling the batter into balls, and then rolling each on a clean table. Press the two ends together to form a tater tot shape, more squared off on the ends.
7. Heat oil in a cast iron skillet, set over medium heat. Upon frying the tater tots, reduce the heat to medium-low. Fry 6 to 9 pieces at a time, while flipping as they crisp on each side. Lay each cooked tater tot on a paper towel to cool.

Yield: 4 x 9-pc servings

Nutritional values per serving:
249 Calories | 21g Fats | 4g Net Carbohydrates | 10.3g Protein

Kale Sprout Fries

Ingredients:
½-bag kale sprouts
2-tbsp parmesan cheese
Salt and pepper to taste
Oil for deep-frying
Directions:
1. Heat the oil in a deep fat fryer.
2. Place the kale sprouts in the fryer basket without overcrowding inside.
3. Fry the kale sprouts until browned on the edges of the bulb, and dark green on the leaves.
4. After frying, place the fries on paper towels to drain excess grease.
5. Sprinkle salt, pepper and parmesan cheese.

Yield: 2-servings
Nutritional values per serving:
109 Calories | 8.5g Fats | 1.5g Net Carbohydrates | 4g Protein

Cheesy Broccoli Fritters with Dill and Lemony Mayo Dip

Ingredients:
For the fritters

¾-cup	almond flour
¼-cup + 3-tbsps	flaxseed meal
4-oz	fresh broccoli
4-oz	mozzarella cheese
2-pcs	eggs, large
2-tsps	baking powder

Salt and pepper to taste

For the sauce

¼-cup	mayonnaise
¼-cup	fresh dill, chopped (or 1-tbsp dried dill)
½-tbsp	lemon juice

Salt and pepper to taste

Directions:
For the fritters

1. Put the broccoli in a food processor. Pulse until the broccoli breaks down into small pieces.
2. Combine the cheese, almond flour, flaxseed meal and baking powder with the broccoli. Season the mixture with salt and pepper to taste.
3. Add the eggs and mix well until well combined.
4. Roll the batter into fritters. Coat each ball with flaxseed meal. Set the fritters aside on a paper towel.
5. Heat a deep fat fryer to 375ºF. Lay the cheese and broccoli fritters inside the fryer basket while not overcrowding it.
6. Fry the fritters for about 3 to 5 minutes, or until golden brown. After frying, lay down the fritters on paper towels to drain excess grease.

For the sauce

7. Create a zesty dill and lemon mayonnaise for a dip by combining all the sauce ingredients.

Yield: 16-servings
Nutritional values per serving:
Sans sauce: 78 Calories | 5.8g Fats | 1.3g Net Carbohydrates |
4.6g Protein
With sauce: 101 Calories | 8.3g Fats | 1.3g Net Carbohydrates |
4.6g Protein

Breadsticks

Ingredients:
For the breadstick base

2-cups (*8-oz*)	mozzarella cheese
¾-cup	almond flour
1-tbsp	Psyllium husk powder
3-tbsps (*1.5 oz*)	cream cheese
1-pc	egg, large
1-tsp	baking powder

For the Italian style

2-tbsps	Italian seasoning
1-tsp	salt
1-tsp	pepper

For the extra cheesy

1-tsp	garlic powder
1-tsp	onion powder
3-oz	cheddar cheese
¼-cup	parmesan cheese

For the cinnamon sugar

3-tbsps	butter
6-tbsps	Swerve® sweetener
2-tbsps	cinnamon

Directions:
For the breadstick base
1. Preheat the oven to 400ºF.
2. Combine the egg and cream cheese in a bowl. Set aside.
3. Combine all the dry ingredients, except for the mozzarella cheese, in another bowl.
4. Melt the mozzarella cheese in the microwave with intervals of 20 seconds, stirring the cheese each time you take it out. Continue cooking until sizzling.

5. Combine altogether the egg and cream cheese mixture, and the dry ingredients with the mozzarella cheese. Mix well.
6. Knead the dough with bare hands. Set on a Silpat® non-stick baking mat.
7. Press the dough flat on the baking sheet until covered with dough. Transfer the dough on a foil so that you can cut the dough on it.
8. Cut the dough as per desired size, and season as per ingredients of either, Italian style or extra cheesy or cinnamon sugar.
9. Bake for about 13 to 15 minutes on the oven's top rack until crisp.

Yield: 6 x 4-breadstick servings
Nutritional values per serving:
Italian Style: 238 Calories | 18.8g Fats | 2.6g Net Carbohydrates | 12.8g Protein
Extra Cheesy: 314 Calories | 24.7g Fats | 3.6g Net Carbohydrates | 18g Protein
Cinnamon Sugar: 291.7 Calories | 24.3g Fats | 3.3g Net Carbohydrates | 13g Protein

Malay Begedil Potato Patty

Ingredients:

3.5-oz	rutabaga, sliced
3.5-oz	cauliflower
2-pcs	shallots, small, sliced
4-tbsps	ground beef
1-tbsp	celery leaves, chopped
1-tbsp	green onion, chopped
½-tsp	white pepper (or black pepper)
¼-tsp	salt
1-pc	egg, large
4-tbsps	coconut oil

Directions:

1. Fry the slices of rutabaga in coconut oil until browned.
2. Pound the fried rutabaga using a pestle and mortar until soft. Set aside.
3. Cook the cauliflower in the microwave until soft, and pound it using a pestle and mortar.
4. Fry the sliced shallots with coconut oil in a small and shallow wok until browned and crispy, yet, not burnt. Set aside after cooking.
5. Sauté the ground beef using the same oil for frying the rutabaga slices. Cook until the surfaces are brown. Season it with salt and pepper to taste.
6. Place the pounded rutabaga and cauliflower, fried shallots, sautéed ground beef, celery leaves and green onion, white pepper (or black pepper) and salt in a bowl. Mix well.
7. Shape a small patty out of the mixture by scooping about a tablespoon. Ensure making ten patties.
8. Whisk the egg in another bowl and coat each patty, but not completely, prior to frying each.
9. Fry the patties with coconut oil until brown.

Yield: 10-servings

Nutritional values per serving:
98 Calories | 8.6g Fats | 1g Net Carbohydrates | 1.7g Protein

Brussels Sprouts Au Gratin

Ingredients:
For the Brussels sprouts

6-oz	Brussels sprouts, stems chopped off
1.8-oz	onion, diced
1-tsp	garlic, minced
2-tbsps	butter
1-tbsp	soy sauce
½-tsp	liquid smoke
¼-tsp	pepper

For the cheese sauce

1-tbsp	butter
½-cup	heavy cream
2.5-oz	cheddar cheese, grated
¼-tsp	paprika
¼-tsp	turmeric
¼-tsp	pepper
⅛-tsp	Xanthan gum

For the pork rind crust

0.5-oz	pork rinds
3-tbsps	parmesan cheese
½-tsp	paprika

Directions:
For the Brussels sprouts

1. Preheat oven to 375°F.
2. Melt the butter until browned in a pan, set over high heat. Add the Brussels sprouts and season with pepper. Allow cooking for about 2 to 3 minutes.
3. Add the diced onion and minced garlic. Add the soy sauce and liquid smoke soon as the onions become soft and translucent. Set aside after cooking.
4. Combine heavy cream and butter in a saucepan. Season the mixture with paprika, turmeric, pepper, and Xanthan gum.

Whisk thoroughly in order for the Xanthan gum to start thickening. Add grated cheese to the sauce and stir gradually.
5. Add the Brussels sprouts once the sauce thickens and becomes creamy. Mix well.
6. Separate the mixture into four ramekins.

For the pork rind crust
7. In a spice grinder or food processor, grind pork rinds, parmesan cheese, and paprika. Use the crumbs for toppings.
8. Bake at 375°F for about 17 to 20 minutes, or until the pork rind and parmesan crust are slightly crispy.

Yield: 4-servings
Nutritional values per serving:
303 Calories | 27.3g Fats | 4.5g Net Carbohydrates | 9.5g Protein

Crispy Cauliflower Cake

Ingredients:

16-oz	cauliflower, chopped into florets
3-stalks	spring onion, medium, sliced
3-oz	white cheddar cheese, shredded
½-cup	ground pork rinds (puffy kind)
½-tsp	salt
¾-tsp	pepper
½-tsp	red pepper flakes
½-tsp	tarragon, dried
¼-tsp	garlic powder
3-tbsps	olive oil
1-pc	egg, large
2-tsps	Psyllium husk powder

Directions:

1. Preheat the oven to 400ºF.
2. Place cauliflower florets in a Ziploc® bag, and then add olive oil, salt and pepper. Shake well to coat thoroughly the cauliflower florets.
3. Place the cauliflower florets onto a baking sheet covered with foil, and bake for about 35 minutes.
4. Meanwhile, put the ground pork rinds in a food processor. Grind the pork rinds until turning into a crumbly meal-like texture.
5. Lightly whisk the egg in a bowl, and add spring onions, shredded white cheddar, Psyllium husk powder, black pepper, red pepper flakes, dried tarragon, and garlic powder.
6. After roasting the cauliflower, place it in a food processor, and pulse it for a few times to break the florets up.
7. Combine all the ingredients in the bowl except pork rind crumbs. Mix everything well until a sticky mixture forms.
8. Form the cauliflower mixture into patties, and then dredge in the pork rind crumbs. Repeat to make about 8 patties, and

lay them on the same baking sheet you used to roast the cauliflower.
9. Bake at 400°F for about 25 minutes. For a crispier exterior, broil the patties further for about 2 to 3 minutes.

Yield: 8-servings
Nutritional values per serving:
154 Calories | 11.9g Fats | 1.8g Net Carbohydrates | 6.9g Protein

Roasted Spicy Lemony Broccoli

Ingredients:

1½-lbs	broccoli florets
⅓-cup	parmesan cheese
¼-cup	olive oil
2-tbsps	fresh basil, chopped
3-tsps	garlic, minced
½ to ¾-tsp	kosher salt
½-tsp	red chili flakes

Zest of ½-pc lemon
Juice of ½-pc lemon

Directions:
1. Preheat the oven to 425°F.
2. Arrange broccoli florets onto a baking sheet covered with parchment paper.
3. Season the broccoli with olive oil, chopped fresh basil, minced garlic, kosher salt, red chili flakes, zest and juice of half a lemon each.
4. Sprinkle parmesan cheese over the top of the broccoli and place in the oven to bake for about 20 to 25 minutes.

Yield: 6-servings
Nutritional values per serving:
137 Calories | 10.5g Fats | 3.7g Net Carbohydrates | 5.7g Protein

Goat Cheese Tomato Tart

Ingredients:
For the roasted tomatoes

2-pcs   tomatoes, medium, cut into ¼-inch slices
¼-cup   olive oil
Salt & pepper to taste

For the tart base

½-cup   almond flour
1-tbsp   Psyllium husk powder
2-tbsps   coconut flour
5-tbsps   cold butter, cubed
¼-tsp   salt

For the tart filling

½-pc   onion, medium, sliced thin
3-oz   goat cheese
2-tbsps   olive oil
2-tsps   garlic, minced
3-tsps   fresh thyme

Directions:
For the roasted tomatoes

1. Preheat the oven to 425ºF.
2. Lay the slices of tomatoes on a baking sheet with parchment paper. Drizzle with olive oil and season with salt and pepper to taste. Stab the tomatoes using a toothpick in order for their juice to run out lest causing creases or a steaming effect.
3. Bake the tomatoes for about 30 to 40 minutes, or until roasted and lost most of their juice. Set aside after cooking.

For the tart base

4. Combine almond flour, Psyllium husk powder, cold butter, coconut flour, and salt in a food processor. Gradually pulse the ingredients until dough begins to form.

5. Press the dough into silicone cupcake molds. Ensure these layers are quite thin at about ¼″ to ½″ thick.
6. Switch the oven heat to 350 ºF and bake the tarts for about 17 to 20 minutes, or until golden brown.
7. Turn the silicone cupcake molds upside down, and lightly tap the bottom so that the tart dough falls out.
8. Layer the roasted tomato onto each tart, and set aside.

For the tart filling
9. Caramelize with olive oil the onion and garlic.
10. Add the caramelized onions and garlic on top of the tomato.
11. Sprinkle fresh thyme and crumble goat cheese over each tart
12. Bake for an additional 5 to 6 minutes, or until the cheese begins melting.

Yield: 12-servings
Nutritional values per serving:
162 Calories | 15.6g Fats | 2.1g Net Carbohydrates | 2.8g Protein

Cucumber Salad

Ingredients:

¾-pc	cucumber, large, sliced thinly
1-packet	shirataki noodles
2-tbsps	coconut oil
1-stalk	spring onion, medium
¼-tsp	red pepper flakes

1-tbsp sesame oil
1-tbsp rice vinegar
1-tsp sesame seeds
Salt and pepper to taste

Directions:

1. Rinse the shiritaki noodles thoroughly, ensuring to wash off all of the extra water that comes along in its package.
2. Place noodles on a kitchen towel to absorb the water and dry them.
3. Heat the coconut oil in a pan, set over medium-high heat.
4. Add the dried noodles, and allow frying for about 5 to 7 minutes, or until browned and crisp.
5. After frying, place the shiritaki noodles on new paper towels to cool and dry.
6. Arrange the sliced cucumber on a plate as to your preferential design.
7. Place the shiritaki noodles over the cucumbers, and top it with spring onion, red pepper flakes, sesame oil, rice vinegar, sesame seeds, and salt and pepper to taste.
8. To add a salty component to the dish, you may also pour over the coconut oil from the pan where you fried the noodles.
9. Store the dish in the refrigerator for at least half an hour prior to serving.

Yield: One serving
Nutritional values per serving:
416 Calories | 43g Fats | 7g Net Carbohydrates | 2g Protein

Conclusion

Ketogenic diets relatively emphasize the composition of foods that are rich in natural fats and sufficient in protein, while restricting foods that are high in carbohydrates.

While the standard American diet (SAD) comprises about 45-65% of calories taken from carbohydrates, ketogenic diets limit carbohydrate consumption to only 2-4% of calories.

It is noteworthy that the low-carb ketogenic diet is not a high-protein regimen, contrary to what many people and pseudo-experts think. It is actually a high-fat diet with moderated and regulated protein consumption, and a greatly reduced carbohydrate allowance. A typical ketogenic meal generally consists of small quantities of protein, a source of natural or organic fats and some green leafy vegetables.

The working principle behind the diet is using ketones as a substitute energy source. When digesting foods containing carbohydrates, they are metabolically broken down into glucose in the body. With larger carbohydrate consumptions, blood sugar levels increase, or an occurrence of more glucose.

Diabetics understand that a high blood sugar is dangerous to the body. Consuming more fats and protein and less carbohydrates leads to a shift in our body metabolism, which taps to use our stored fats to convert them into energy in lieu of burning sugar or glucose. The shift produces more ketone bodies, and at the same time, decreases blood sugar levels.

When glucose drops and ketone bodies rise and dominate in the bloodstream, the heart, muscle, brain and other body organs cease to burn sugar. Rather, they use the ketone bodies as an alternative fuel source and nutritional or optimal ketosis is established.

Soon as the body applies ketones as major fuel sources, a wide variety of beneficial effects ensue. A ketone-producing, high fat, low-carb diet is truly great for reducing weight, slowing the aging process and addressing a wide array of health issues.

In fact, ketogenic diets are greatly more powerful than the more popular and trendy regimen would suggest. Both anti-inflammatory and anti-oxidant effects of nutritional ketosis prove to be potent. Currently, medical research and studies still continue to explore more about nutritional or optimal ketosis for further applications and benefits it may bestow to humankind.

Overall, eating a high amount of fat, moderate protein, and low amount of carbs can have a massive impact in your health—lowering your cholesterol, body weight, and blood sugar, while raising your energy and mood levels. Indeed, being under the state of ketosis can certainly alleviate and augment in the treatment of several serious health issues.

As a summary, the ketogenic diet is neither a trend nor a current fad. It is a powerful regulator of metabolic disorders. When implemented properly, it is capable of being extremely effective. The bottom line for ketogenic diets is how you can enhance or increase your energy levels and improve your health by simply altering the way you eat.

Free Ebook Offer

The Ultimate Guide To Vitamins

I'm very excited to be able to make this offer to you. This is a wonderful 10k word ebook that has been made available to you through my publisher, Valerian Press. As a health conscious person you should be well aware of the uses and health benefits of each of the vitamins that should make up our diet. This book gives you an easy to understand, scientific explanation of the vitamin followed by the recommended daily dosage. It then highlights all the important health benefits of each vitamin. A list of the best sources of each vitamin is provided and you are also given some actionable next steps for each vitamin to make sure you are utilizing the information!

As well as receiving the free ebooks you will also be sent a weekly stream of free ebooks, again from my publishing company Valerian Press. You can expect to receive at least a new, free ebook each and every week. Sometimes you might receive a massive 10 free books in a week!

All you need to do is simply type this link into your browser: http://bit.ly/18hmup4

About The Author

Hi, I'm Martin Rowland! Thanks for visiting my page, if you have read any of my books I sincerely hope they brought a lot of value into your life. If you haven't, what are you waiting for! A life full of health, energy and abundance await you, should you apply that you learn from my books. Clean Eating is my absolute passion, ever since I took the plunge a few years back my life has been phenomenal. I have competed in marathons, seen my abs for the very first time and completely transformed my mental health. When I meet people who haven't seen me since my transformation they are stunned. It's all down to clean eating.

Outside of writing and passionately preaching about clean diets I like to spend my time reading great fiction. I can often be found spending entire weekends sitting next to the lake beside my house engrossed in a novel. It has taken me a long time to get around to it, but I am finally enjoying the wonderful work that is George Martins' A Song of Ice and Fire series. Isn't it just brilliant? My other favourite thing to do is sailing. On the weekends where you can't find me beside the lake I will be cruising along the south coast on my wonderful yacht 'Poppy'.

Valerian Press

At Valerian Press we have three key beliefs.

Providing outstanding value: We believe in enriching all of our customers' lives, doing everything we can to ensure the best experience.

Championing new talent: We believe in showcasing the worlds emerging talent by giving them the platform to grow.

Simplicity and efficiency: We understand how valuable your time is. Our products are stream-lined and consist only of what you want. You will find no fluff with us.

We hope you have enjoyed reading Martins guide to the Ketogenic Diet!

We would love to offer you a regular supply of our free and discounted books. We cover a huge range of non-fiction genres; diet and cookbooks, health and fitness, alternative and holistic medicine, spirituality and plenty more. All you need to do is type this link into your web browser: http://bit.ly/18hmup4

20353155R00073

Printed in Great Britain
by Amazon